Immunochemical Methods in the Biological Sciences: Enzymes and Proteins

BIOLOGICAL TECHNIQUES SERIES

J. E. TREHERNE
Department of Zoology
University of Cambridge
England

P. H. RUBERY
Department of Biochemistry
University of Cambridge
England

1. Ion-sensitive Intracellular Microelectrodes, *R. C. Thomas* 1978
2. Time-lapse Cinemicroscopy, *P. N. Riddle* 1979
3. Immunochemical Methods in the Biological Sciences: Enzymes and Proteins, *R. J. Mayer and J. H. Walter,* 1980

Immunochemical Methods in the Biological Sciences: Enzymes and Proteins

R. J. Mayer
Senior Lecturer, Department of Biochemistry,
University of Nottingham Medical School,
Queen's Medical Centre, Clifton Boulevard,
Nottingham, NG7 2UH, UK

and

J. H. Walker
Research Fellow, Abteilung für Neurochemie,
Max Planck Institut für Biophysikalische Chemie,
Göttingen-Nikolausberg, Göttingen, GFR

ACADEMIC PRESS
A Subsidiary of Harcourt Brace Jovanovich
London · New York · Toronto · Sydney · San Francisco

ACADEMIC PRESS INC. (LONDON) LTD
24/28 Oval Road
London NW1

United States Edition published by
ACADEMIC PRESS INC.
111 Fifth Avenue
New York, New York 10003

British Cataloguing in Publication Data
Mayer, R D
　　Immunochemical methods in the biological sciences. –
　　(Biological techniques series).
　　1. Enzymes　2. Immunochemistry – Technique
　　3. Proteins
　　I. Title　II. Walker, J H　III. Series
　　574.1'925　QP601　80–40297

　　ISBN 0–12–480750–X

Printed in Great Britain by
The Pitman Press, Bath

Preface

We would not have been stimulated to write this book without the excitement of using immunochemical techniques in the authors' laboratories. The excitement was often provided by the "unsung heroes" who helped to carry out many of the techniques. We therefore gratefully acknowledge the co-operation and skills of Ron, Linda, Janice, Janet, Elaine, Susan, Rowland, Ray, Reg, Alex, Pete, Trevor, Brian, Sue, Norman, Khalidah, Patrick and Jenny. We would like to thank Dr Colin Wild for indexing the book.

February, 1980   R. J. Mayer
                                                                               J. H. Walker

To the late Professor G. H. A. Hübscher, Foundation Professor in Biochemistry, University of Nottingham Medical School, Nottingham, UK

Contents

4
Uses of Antisera

5
**Case Study I: Immunochemical Studies on Membrane
Protein Antigens**

1
Introduction

I. General Introduction

The science of biochemistry can be distinguished, perhaps aphoristically, from chemistry by the way in which enzymes bring about what are otherwise thermodynamically unfavourable chemical reactions. Since it is also axiomatic that enzymes are proteins it is not surprising that many years of dedication have been devoted to the determination of protein structure and function: indeed, much of the last 20 years in biochemistry has been devoted to such studies and remarkable advances have been made, not least in the elucidation of the structures of the immunoglobulins themselves. Latterly more emphasis has been placed on studies of the ways in which enzyme activity can be regulated *in vitro* and particularly *in vivo*: here normal physiological control of enzyme activity has been resolved into rapid (acute) and slow (chronic) mechanisms. Acute regulation of enzyme activity is carried out without altering the amount of the particular regulatory enzyme(s), whereas chronic regulation is achieved by changing the amount(s) of key regulatory enzymes. Not only have the normal physiological regulators been defined (e.g. hormones), but also the effect of a large variety of exogenous agents has been studied. It can safely be said that, with a few very rare exceptions, the broad division into acute and chronic changes in enzyme activity and therefore physiological regulation of metabolism has been defined, and can only be further elaborated, by means of immunochemical techniques. The only satisfactory straightforward way to measure the amount of an enzyme or protein in a tissue extract is by means of these techniques. Chronic changes in enzyme or protein amounts in response to a variety of stimuli have, therefore, been shown predominantly by immunochemical methods.

1

Interestingly immunoisolation of enzymes or proteins from tissue extracts is the method of choice for many workers in the field of acute enzyme regulation. Here changes in enzyme activity are often mediated by protein modification (e.g. phosphorylation): antibodies can therefore be very effectively used to make the rapid isolation of modified species, which is needed in order to establish the extent of modification in different physiological or pathological states.

Studies of enzymes and proteins throughout the animal and plant kingdoms can be very effectively carried out immunochemically. It is salutory that interpretation of any work on physiological or pathological changes in enzyme activity in a tissue will ultimately hang on whether the amount or just the activity of an enzyme changes; this can only be effectively resolved immunochemically. Immunochemical reagents are being increasingly used for cell and molecular biological purposes. Enzymes and proteins in a variety of cell membranes and organelles are being probed immunochemically. These studies are leading to substantial advances in our understanding of membrane structure, function and turnover. Eventually biological scientists must ask if they can afford *not* to use immunochemical techniques.

Perhaps not surprisingly the greatest sympathy for these biological problems comes from biologists and not immunologists; a consequence of this is that the biologists must perfect the skills and techniques, albeit often established in principle by immunologists, to solve their specific problems in immunochemistry. The work described in this book is a personal account of an attempt made by two biochemists to grasp and solve many of the immunochemical problems which are routinely presented to biologists. As usual in science it is not that the techniques are not available but that the scientists studying particular scientific problems are not aware of them; alternatively designers of techniques do not know of all the uses to which their methods may be put. Scientific developments in a field are ultimately entwined in the scientific philosophy of their perpetrators. This is often overlooked and can be reduced to the desire to understand some particular scientific problem. Biochemistry is fundamental to all biological sciences and, therefore, this book is written for all biologists who may wish to start an immunochemical study of enzymes or proteins from scratch; it does not catalogue all the available techniques in immunology but tries to emphasize the developmental sequence of methods and techniques which can convert any biologist into a practising immunochemist.

II. Aims and Objectives

Immunochemistry is the study of the interaction between antigens (e.g.

proteins) and antibodies. Immunization of an animal produces antibodies against proteins which the animal recognizes to be "foreign". The immunoglobulins which are produced in response to this challenge are specific to the antigen (or antigens) injected. The immunoglobulin population which is specific to an antigen is heterogeneous, in that subpopulations of immunoglobulin exist which interact with different regions (or antigenic determinants) on the surface of the antigen.

A problem in writing a book on this topic is that there is a tendency to generalize about immunochemical processes which are by definition not general but very specific phenomena. The production, processing and use of each antiserum will vary depending on the antigen of interest. Furthermore biologists have very different interests in the properties of enzymes and proteins and, therefore, the requirements and objectives of each research group will be different. Naturally this will lead to the use of different methods for the identification, isolation and quantitation of antigens from tissue extracts: the purity of antibodies needed for a piece of work may vary from crude antiserum (e.g. for immunotitration of enzyme activity) to carefully purified antibodies (for immunoadsorbent chromatography or antigen quantitation). Potential immunochemists should consider their specific requirements carefully before choosing from the methods and procedures which are outlined in this book.

Immunochemical studies (with humoral antibodies, i.e. in the serum) have been carried out on enzyme activity, enzyme evolution, the nature of antigenic determinants on enzymes, immunogenicity in relation to enzyme structure and function, the relationship between proenzymes and enzymes and between apoenzymes and enzymes, multiple forms of enzymes and allostery. The results indicate the complex relationship between factors responsible for immunogenicity of a protein antigen, e.g. level of conformational organization, and the subsequent interaction of antibodies with the protein antigen (Arnon, 1973).

Sensitive immunochemical techniques are being used increasingly to measure the amount and rate of turnover (synthesis and degradation) of enzymes and proteins (Philippidis et al., 1972; Speake et al., 1976). Immunochemical methods have recently been developed to isolate polyribosomes containing immunoreactive nascent antigen chains, from which specific mRNA can be prepared (Palacios et al., 1972).

Naturally there are difficulties in carrying out immunochemical studies on proteins and enzymes. Problems arise not only in connection with methodology but also in relation to the interpretation of experimental data, e.g. reactions of identity with unstable proteins or membrane proteins.

The purpose of this book is to review the methods involved in the production, processing and use of antisera to proteins and enzymes. Each section is structured to emphasize the principles, practice, generality and problems of each technique. The book is not intended as a completely comprehensive guide to all immunochemical techniques which have been used to study proteins or enzymes. Such studies have been reviewed (Cinader, 1963, 1967; Clausen, 1971; Arnon, 1971, 1973; Kwapinski, 1972; Bjerrum and Bøg-Hansen, 1976b). The book is intended to be a practical guide to anyone wishing to raise and use antisera to proteins or enzymes. It is hoped that the contents will be useful to those involved in a study of soluble or membrane protein antigens in any biological system. The book is based in part on the authors' immunochemical studies of fatty-acid synthetase (Speake et al., 1975, 1976), acetyl-CoA carboxylase (Manning et al., 1976), 6-phosphogluconate dehydrogenase (Betts and Mayer, 1975, 1977), cytochrome oxidase (Walker and Mayer, 1976), monoamine oxidase (Dennick and Mayer, 1977), casein (Al-Sarraj et al., 1978) and cholinergic vesicle proteins. The studies are related to the turnover of the named enzymes (Walker et al., 1976) and the cholinergic mechanism of nervous transmission respectively.

2

Antiserum Production

Antisera may be produced against a single protein antigen (monospecific antiserum) or against a mixture of protein antigens (polyspecific or multispecific antiserum). For many immunochemical studies on enzymes or proteins it is advantageous to produce a monospecific antiserum (Walker *et al.*, 1976). However, polyspecific antisera may be produced deliberately to analyse complex protein mixtures (Bjerrum and Bøg-Hansen, 1976a). Alternatively, an antiserum may be raised to an antigen of interest prepared from a species which is not to be studied (e.g. beef heart cytochrome c oxidase has been used to raise an antiserum which was used to study the rat liver enzyme, Hackenbrock and Hammon, 1975; bovine dopamine β-hydroxylase has been used to raise an antiserum to study the rat brain enzyme, Ross *et al.*, 1978). Furthermore antisera may be prepared to commercially available antigens (e.g. Glutamine synthetase, Koch and Nielsen, 1975) although it is advisable to test the purity of the antigen before beginning the immunization schedule. Such an assessment may indicate that further purification of an antigen is necessary before immunization can be started.

I. Preparation of Antigens

A. Antigen Purity

As a working principle it should always be assumed that an antigen which is pure by biochemical criteria (e.g. single component in protein analytical systems) is not pure immunologically. This assumption can avoid tremendous disappointment after a lengthy immunization schedule. There are many examples of biochemically pure antigens giving rise to polyspecific antisera (Clausen, 1971) and in our own laboratory only one protein antigen (fatty acid synthetase) out of many has given rise to a monospecific antiserum.

The major dilemma for the enzymologist is to decide how far to purify the antigen, measured in terms of time and effort, given that there are a variety of procedures for antiserum purification (Chapter 3), and that however hard he tries his antigen may still be impure. As usual, experience is the only guide, but in general it is best to obtain the most purified preparation for use as antigen, knowing that the antiserum can subsequently be purified if necessary.

B. *Nature of Antigen Preparation*

Enzyme and protein purification procedures give rise to preparations in buffer solutions of different pH and ionic strength which can contain a variety of agents which have been included to protect the protein from inactivation (e.g. dithiothreitol, 2-mercaptoethanol, EDTA, glycerol, stabilizing ions and coenzymes). Work with membrane protein antigens usually means the isolation and purification of a protein in the presence of detergents (often non-ionic) or at very high salt concentrations (e.g. 3 M KCl for plasma membrane antigens, Price and Baldwin, 1977). These agents may affect the microheterogeneity of antibody subpopulations (e.g. by masking antigenic determinants), but in general there is little evidence that they affect antibody production. Antisera to membrane antigens in detergents (e.g. Triton X-100) are not difficult to produce (e.g. Dennick and Mayer, 1977).

Although ionic detergents (e.g. sodium dodecyl sulphate) are known to disrupt antigen–antibody interactions (Crumpton and Parkhouse, 1972; Bjerrum and Bøg-Hansen, 1976b) antisera have been successfully raised to protein subunits isolated by polyacrylamide gel electrophoresis in the presence of sodium dodecyl sulphate. For example, Strauss *et al.* (1975) homogenized antigen-containing gel in phosphate-buffered saline and injected it into rabbit foot pads. Similarly immunization with single bands obtained by polyacrylamide gel electrophoresis in the presence of sodium dodecyl sulphate has been successfully used to raise monospecific antisera to actin (Blomberg *et al.*, 1977), microtubule associated protein (Sherline and Schiavone, 1977) and myosin (Tashiro and Stadtler, personal communication). It must be remembered that polypeptides of similar molecular weight may be present in a single piece (band) of polyacrylamide gel, e.g. tubulin and a polypeptide associated with neurofilaments (Gilbert,1978). However, immunization with antigens prepared in this way has great potential for membrane antigens which are often very difficult to resolve, purify and identify in systems which do not contain sodium dodecyl sulphate. Protein subunits prepared in sodium dodecyl sulphate will more frequently be used as antigens, as more laboratories use two dimensional polyacrylamide gel electrophoresis to purify membrane protein subunits (Dale and Latner, 1969; O'Farrell, 1975). It is often easier to prepare a protein subunit reproducibly by these methods than to try and purify native proteins from some cellular organelle (e.g. synaptic vesicle membrane proteins).

It is tempting to suggest that all so-called purified proteins should be subjected to polyacrylamide gel electrophoresis in the presence of sodium dodecyl sulphate; following staining the subunit or subunits of the antigen of interest could be cut out, pooled and used for the preparation of samples for immunization. This approach could minimize the production of antibodies to contaminating antigens, except, of course, to those contaminants which have the same subunit size(s) as the antigen of interest. Excellent antiserum to human liver monoamine oxidase has recently been produced in this way (Russell et al., 1978a).

However, the problems of interpretation associated with the use of antisera to subunits of functional protein complexes in membranes must be recognized. For example antisera raised to subunits isolated from multi-subunit enzyme complexes may not cross-react with the holoenzyme (Werner, 1974).

C. Antigen Mixtures

Many polyspecific antisera have been prepared to protein mixtures and have been used to identify and quantify soluble (e.g. Weeke, 1973b) and membrane (e.g. Bjerrum and Bøg-Hansen, 1976a) antigens. Polyspecific antisera can be used to study qualitative and quantitative changes in antigen populations (e.g. in membrane fusion or during chronic enzyme adaptation in tissues).

If the resolution of crossed-rocket immunoelectrophoresis is sufficiently good, immunoprecipitates can be cut from the agarose gel and used to produce monospecific antisera (Koch and Nielsen, 1975). However, it is very useful to be able to identify the biochemical nature of the antigen in a particular immunoprecipitate if the subsequent monospecific antiserum is to be of maximal use in biological experiments. Identification of an enzyme which retains activity in an immunoprecipitate is relatively simple (Blomberg and Perlman, 1971a; Clausen, 1971). Similarly, proteins which bind calcium (Suttie et al., 1977), epinephrine (Blomberg and Berzins, 1975), or which are phosphorylated (Gordon et al., 1977) are easy to identify in immunoprecipitates after the incorporation of radio-labelled ligand or through change in the electrophoretic mobility of the antigens after binding of the ligand. Identification of enzymically inactive antigens in immunoprecipitates can be difficult and equivocal and, paradoxically, often requires the use of purified antigen to identify the rocket immunoprecipitate of interest. However, the increasing number of methods which are becoming available to characterize antigens in immunoprecipitates (Chapter 4) will make this problem much simpler.

The relative immunogenicities of proteins in a mixture are of great importance when considering the outcome of an immunization schedule designed to obtain a polyspecific antiserum. The problem is that some proteins may be much better macromolecular antigens than others, thus complicating the subsequent use of the antiserum (e.g. in immunoprecipitation analyses in gels).

Indeed, in some cases it may not be possible to obtain precipitating antibodies to some of the major protein species in an antigen mixture, while minor protein species may give rise to high titres of antibodies (e.g. in cholinergic synaptic vesicles). It may be that a single protein in a protein mixture may be the only effective antigen in the mixture. Injection of whole chromaffin granules seems to give rise to a monospecific antiserum to dopamine β-hydroxylase (Helle et al., 1979).

When preparing polyspecific antisera to membrane antigens, contaminating cytosolic proteins may act as excellent antigens giving much better antibody production than the membrane antigens. Furthermore, even when the intention is to produce a monospecific antiserum (e.g. to purified integral mitochondrial membrane enzymes) contaminants in the preparations can give much larger titres of antibodies than the antigens of interest (e.g. Walker et al., 1976; Dennick and Mayer, unpublished data).

II. Preparation of Antigens for Immunization

A. Adjuvants

Protein antigens are usually mixed with material that will increase the concentration of circulating antibodies, i.e. adjuvants. There are a variety of adjuvants which may themselves be antigenic (e.g. tubercle bacilli) or not (mineral oil) but which can improve the humoral immune response by mechanisms which include increasing the number of cells involved in antibody formation, assuring a more efficient processing of antigens and prolonging the duration of the antigen in the immunized animal. The most commonly used adjuvant is complete Freund's adjuvant, which consists of killed mycobacteria (e.g. tubercle bacilli), an oil and an emulsifier. In incomplete Freund's adjuvant the mycobacteria are omitted (Clausen, 1971). Many immunization schedules for proteins have been used but they differ in that some authors prefer to use Freund's complete adjuvant for the first series of injections and subsequently use incomplete adjuvant (e.g. Mason *et al.*, 1973), whereas other authors prefer to use complete adjuvant throughout (e.g. Walker *et al.*, 1976). The disadvantage of using complete adjuvant throughout an immunization schedule is that sterile abscesses can be produced by subcutaneous but not intramuscular injections. In the authors' experience approximately 20–30% of animals (rabbits or sheep) may develop such abscesses, which can be treated effectively by topical application of anti-inflammatory agents.

Equal volumes of the antigen preparation and the adjuvant are vigorously mixed to give a stable emulsion which can be used as the preparation for injection. A stable emulsion may be produced by repeated aspiration of the mixture into and out of a hypodermic syringe with a large gauge needle, by homogenization with a loose-fitting pestle or by sonication. Recently a synthetic adjuvant, moramyl dipeptide, has become available (Institut Pasteur). This compound apparently possesses several advantages over Freund's adjuvant, including an increased ability to induce the humoral immune response. Precipitation of antigens onto aluminium oxide is also frequently used to immobilize antigens (Hudson and Hay, 1976). Samples of *Bordatella pertassis* may be added to enhance the immune response.

B. Amount of Antigen

Humoral antibody production is a function of the nature (e.g. with or without adjuvant) and amount of the antigen and the immune response of the individual animal. A poor immune response (immune tolerance) can occur to small or large amounts of an antigen (Mitchison, 1968). Enzymologists and protein chemists are often faced with the problem of obtaining enough of their purified protein for biochemical analysis. Fortunately this does not present a problem immunologically where the small amounts of protein antigens available may be quite adequate. For example, excellent precipitating titres have been obtained in sheep with a total of 400 μg of acetyl-CoA carboxylase (Walker *et al.*, 1976). Minute amounts of protein antigens have been used to raise antisera. The fact that antisera have been raised to immunoprecipitates cut out from agarose gels testifies to the sensitivity of the immune response. Similarly, very small amounts of antigen protein (e.g. 1 μg) bound to solid supports will give rise to antisera (Stevenson, 1974). In general, however, a total of 0·5–4·0 mg of protein per rabbit and 1–10 mg of protein per sheep over the entire immunization schedule is recommended. For polyspecific antisera the upper limits of antigen amount suggested above are probably preferable, although it must be stressed that there is no definite answer to the question of how much antigen should be used in an immunization schedule.

C. Weakly Immunogenic Antigens

Some proteins are poor antigens, particularly those which show little evolutionary divergence between mammalian species (e.g. cytochrome c, actin, myosin). Two different approaches have been used to improve the immune response of these proteins. Antisera may be raised to poor mammalian antigens in non-mammals (e.g. myosin in fowl). Alternatively proteins may be modified in some way to improve their immunogenicity. This may be achieved by cross-linking with glutaraldehyde to give homo-polymers (Avrameas and Ternynck, 1969) or heteropolymers (e.g. casein with ovalbumin, Houdebine and Gaye, 1976; S–100 protein with methy-lated bovine serum albumin, Levine, 1967).

Animal caseins are considered poor antigens and the heteropolymeriza-tion procedure described above has been used coupled with prolonged immunization schedules to obtain reasonable precipitating titres. Recently, in our laboratory, a novel technique has been used to obtain excellent precipitating titres against rabbit casein polypeptides (12 mg) in 8–12 weeks in sheep (Al-Sarraj et al., 1978). The preparation for immunization contained Sepharose 2B-albumin-casein. Albumin was linked to Sepharose 2B by a cyanogen bromide procedure (Porath et al., 1973) and casein polypeptides were linked to the Sepharose-albumin with glutaraldehyde (Fig. 1).

It is intriguing that antibodies to albumin are not produced by this procedure: in fact an ideal situation occurs in which the immunogenicity of casein is increased dramatically, whereas that of albumin is apparently abolished. The question arises as to the generality of this phenomenon and to the immunological reasons for the observations.

It has been reported previously (Orlov and Gurvich, 1971) that the immunization of animals with protein-Sephadex complex elicits large quantities of antibodies. Antibody quantities of 10–20 times that seen with the unconjugated protein were observed in the secondary response to antigen. These authors commented that subcutaneous administration was preferred and that no antibodies were produced against Sephadex. Recent-ly attempts have been carried out to raise large titres to bovine brain choline acetylase transferase coupled to Sepharose-albumin in rabbits; little success was achieved in this case (Walker and Mayer, unpublished data). In the small number of cases studied, therefore, coupling of antigens

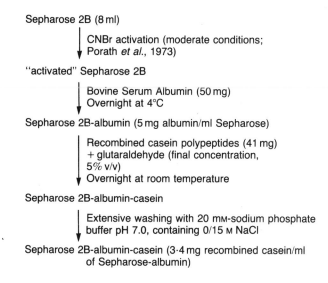

Sepharose 2B (8 ml)

⎮ CNBr activation (moderate conditions;
↓ Porath et al., 1973)

"activated" Sepharose 2B

⎮ Bovine Serum Albumin (50 mg)
↓ Overnight at 4°C

Sepharose 2B-albumin (5 mg albumin/ml Sepharose)

⎮ Recombined casein polypeptides (41 mg)
⎮ + glutaraldehyde (final concentration,
⎮ 5% v/v)
↓ Overnight at room temperature

Sepharose 2B-albumin-casein

⎮ Extensive washing with 20 mM-sodium phosphate
↓ buffer pH 7.0, containing 0/15 M NaCl

Sepharose 2B-albumin-casein (3·4 mg recombined casein/ml
of Sepharose-albumin)

Fig. 1. Preparation of sepharose-albumin-casein.

to Sephadex or Sepharose has sometimes resulted in excellent or limited success. Further investigations of the immunological reasons for this enhanced antibody production need to be carried out.

Conversely, many workers are trying to reduce or abolish the immunogenicity of enzymes in order to use them in enzyme-replacement therapy. Here studies have been carried out with protein heteropolymers where the enzyme (e.g. pig liver uricase) was coupled to homologous rabbit albumin for injection into rabbits. The heteropolymer in these conditions was found to be non-immunogenic and non-antigenic (Remy and Poznansky, 1978). Alternatively, immunogenicity of bovine serum albumin and bovine liver catalase has been abolished in rabbits by coupling of these proteins to polyethylene glycols (Abuchowski et al., 1977a, b). These authors envisage that the linear, flexible, uncharged hydrophilic polymers which are attached to the proteins may abolish immunogenicity by providing a shell around the enzyme that covers antigenic determinants; by presenting a flexible, unbranched hydrophilic surface for inspection by the immune process the interiorized enzyme may not be recognized as a foreign substance.

Such a hypothesis (i.e. burying of protein in dextran or agarose matrix) may also partly explain why no antibodies to bovine serum albumin were obtained in sheep (Al-Sarraj et al., 1978) by injection of Sepharose-albumin-protein. Clearly the reasons for increasing or decreasing the immunogenicity of proteins are not understood; but both objectives are laudable in that increasing immunogenicity is of paramount importance to the immunochemist and abolition of immunogenicity obligatory for enzyme replacement therapy in inborn errors of metabolism.

In principle, however, it should be possible to obtain antibodies to any protein by presenting it to the animal in an immunogenic form. Since antibodies can be obtained to many small molecules (e.g. acetylcholine, Spector *et al.*, 1978) and a wide variety of biologically active compounds (Yalow, 1978), it seems likely that antibodies could be obtained to all proteins, e.g. by careful choice of species for immunization. Some poor protein antigens may behave as haptens, with antibodies only produced against a single antigenic determinant. In such cases the antibodies may only be detectable by immunoaffinity or immunofluorescent techniques.

Finally, it is possible that for some antigens a very long immunization schedule is required before antibodies may be detected (e.g. choline acetyltransferase, Rossier, 1975).

III. Immunization Procedures

A. Selection of Species

Rabbits, goats, sheep and fowl are commonly used for antisera production. Naturally the best antisera are raised in a species which is unrelated to the species from which the antigen was prepared. It should be remembered that the immune response will vary from animal to animal in a given species. This consideration may be important if the antigenicity of a protein is unknown or known to be poor. In such a case it may be better to inject several rabbits instead of one sheep in order to be able to use the best antiserum produced. This approach presumes that sufficient antigen is available for multiple immunization schedules.

Several other considerations affect the choice of species for immunization including expense of animals, housing of animals, source of antigen, volumes of antiserum required (e.g. very large volumes (1 litre) can be obtained in a single bleed from a goat or sheep), and ease of bleeding.

B. Sites of Immunization

Antigen preparations may be presented to animals by several routes. Antigen–adjuvant mixtures may be injected subcutaneously and intramuscularly. Antigen may be injected intravenously or into foot pads (e.g. of rabbits) and in these cases complete Freund's adjuvant may be injected separately at subcutaneous sites (Clausen, 1971). There are two distinct types of immunization procedures: single-site injections and multisite injections. Multisite injections can be given both subcutaneously and intramuscularly, and offer the advantage of presenting the antigen by a variety of routes with the expectation of provoking the maximum immune response. It may be advantageous to immunize rabbits intradermally in the thicker part of the skin above the scapulae (Harboe and Ingild, 1973).

C. Immunization Schedules

Animals should be bled before immunization to obtain non-immune (control) serum. Many types of immunization schedules have been attempted, but in principle antigen is presented at regular intervals on several occasions with trial bleeding after the second and subsequent injections. Details of these procedures are given in the Technical Supplement (Chapter 7).

IV. Trial and Preparative Bleeding Procedures

The methods for carrying out these bleeding procedures are described in detail in the Technical Supplement (Chapter 7). Procedures for the bleeding of rabbits and sheep (also suitable for goats) are described in detail.

V. Monoclonal Antibodies

Classical immunization procedures produce antisera which contain a small proportion of specific immunoglobulin to the antigen of interest mixed with a relatively enormous amount of non-specific immunoglobulins which were present in the animal before commencement of the immunization schedule. It is difficult to estimate the percentage of specific antibodies to an antigen of interest, since this will depend on the specific interactions of the antigen with an animal's immune system. Specific antibodies to a macromolecular antigen of interest may be purified by immunoaffinity methods (see Chapter 4) and by this procedure, for example, it is possible to estimate that approximately 1% of the immunoglobulin G in a sheep immunized extensively with casein, are specific antibodies to casein (Al-Sarraj et al., 1978). The percentage of immunoglobulin which is specific for an antigen of interest can only be estimated by similar immunoadsorption methods. Immunoaffinity purification of antibodies to an antigen of interest must be recommended, since the purified specific antibodies are much more useful than crude antisera for a variety of immunochemical techniques (see Chapter 4).

The objective of immunization with enzymes or proteins is to prepare immunochemical reagents of defined purity and specificity which can be used for a variety of biochemical measurements. Reproducibility is of obvious importance if large numbers of tests are to be carried out with specific antibodies: this may be difficult, if not impossible, if repeated booster immunization of an animal is required in order to obtain sufficient quantity of antiserum. Both the quantity and quality of the antibodies may change during repeated immunization which means that each batch of serum must be carefully assessed and purified before use as an immunochemical reagent. Conventional antibody production is therefore complicated by the inherent variability of biological systems. Naturally all potential users of antisera would be delighted if some or all of this variability could be removed by some improvement in antibody production, as long as one set of biological variables were not replaced by another. The ultimate objective would be the production of large quantities of specific antibody to a single determinant on a macromolecular antigen, although many biologists would settle for specific antibodies to a single macromolecule which would suffice for a number of immunochemical assays. Milstein has provided methods which go a long way towards achieving this goal through somatic cell hybridization techniques.

The principle of the method depends on fusing myeloma cells (having vigorous proliferative capacity in cell culture) to spleen cells from an immunized animal, thus generating hybrid cells which thrive in tissue culture and produce specific antibodies to the antigen of interest. Careful selection of cells which produce specific antibody to antigen of interest can be carried out. Subsequent large scale culture of these cells can lead to the production of enormous quantities of monoclonal antibody which could be used to standardize assays throughout the world, and should avoid the problems involved and time required in purifying specific antibody from the serum of hyper-immunized animals.

The development of these techniques involved the production of hybrid cells which secrete antibodies to sheep red blood cells (Köhler and Milstein, 1975, 1976). Subsequently Milstein and colleagues succeeded in obtaining hybrid cells which produce antibodies to the major histocompatibility antigens (Galfre et al., 1977). The implications of the latter studies for tissue typing before surgical transplantation studies in man are obvious. General outlines of the procedures are described in Tables 1 and 2 and will be analysed in some detail to illustrate some of the methods involved.

Spleen cells from immunized animals (mice or rats) can be fused to an 8-azaguanine-resistant clone of MOPC 21 mouse myeloma cells (BALB/C

Table 1
Protocol for myeloma-spleen cell hybridization

Immunization

Immunize the donor animal intraperitoneally with antigen of interest (1–2 months).

Prepare spleen cell suspension.

Hybridization

Wash spleen cell suspension (approx. 10^7 cells) and 9-azaguanine resistant myeloma cell suspension (approx. 10^7–10^8 cells) at room temperature in Earle's balanced salt solution.

Sediment cells, pool cells, and resuspended in cooled salt solution containing Sendai virus (or Polyethylene glycol).

Incubate at 37°C for 30 min, wash with Dulbecco's modified medium containing 20% horse serum and separate into required number of samples.

Hybrid cell selection

One day after fusion cells are transferred to HAT medium (Hypoxanthine, Aminopterin, Thymidine; Littlefield, 1964). Medium changed at 1–3 day intervals. Aminopterin omitted after 8–14 days. After 4 weeks hybrid cells transferred to ordinary tissue culture conditions.

Table 2
Protocol for clonal selection

Cloning Hybrid cells are cloned in soft Agar and after clones have reached required size.

Selection of antibody secreting cells

Either by Clone plaques in soft Agar
i.e. overlay in sterile conditions with 0·6% Agarose in phosphate-buffered saline containing cells with antigen(s) of interest; fresh guinea pig serum (adsorbed with cells of interest) as souce of complement. Incubate overnight at 37°C. Pick out positive clones and grow large batches in suspension culture.

or by carrying out tests on clone supernatants
i.e. clone cells in soft Agar; pick out individual clones of cells and grow as separate colonies in suspension culture. Take supernatants from clones and test for immunoreactivity (e.g. Chromium[51] release test, immunofluorescence or radioimmune assay). Grow up large batches of positive clones in suspension culture.

Cloned cells which produce specific antibody to antigen of interest can be stored, when necessary, at liquid N_2 temperature.

---

origin). Spleen cells have been fused with secreting (X63-Ag8) and non-secreting variants (NSI/-Ag4-1) of the myeloma cells. The latter cells were chosen to avoid the presence of parental myeloma chains in the hybrids: this obviates the necessity for clonal screening procedures to derive sublines, which only express the antibody-specific L and H chain combination. The defects of the non-secreting parent do not hinder the expression of the second parental immunoglobulin. Furthermore, fusion does not restore the expression of the lost immunoglobulin chains (Köhler and Milstein, 1976).

The general procedures for immunization of the spleen-donor, hybridization of the spleen and myeloma cells, and selection of hybrid cells from unfused myeloma cells and spleen cells is shown in Table 1. Immunization schedules vary but will be of sufficient duration to ensure a good splenic population of plasma cells secreting antibody to the antigen of interest (1–2 months, Köhler and Milstein, 1976). Hybridization of myeloma and spleen cells was initially accomplished with the Sendai virus (Köhler and Milstein, 1975, 1976) but the use of polyethylene glycol as the fusigenic agent is now becoming the method of choice (Galfre et al., 1977). Hybrid cells are initially selected by the fact that they do not die in HAT medium, whereas the myeloma cells, and spleen cells from the immunized animal do not grow in these conditions (Köhler and Milstein, 1975). After growth in the hybrid selection medium cells are transferred to ordinary tissue culture conditions.

Hybrid cells are cloned in soft Agar (Table 2) and colonies secreting antibodies to antigen of interest can be identified directly on the soft Agar plates by means of overlay techniques: individual clones can also be grown in suspension culture and the culture supernatants tested for antibodies to the antigen of interest by a variety of techniques. Positive clones can be grown on a large scale in suspension cultures. Before cloning individual cultures may gradually lose activity whereas others may retain or even increase their antibody secreting activity (Galfre et al., 1977). This presumably reflects the complexity of the cultures: after a time the fastest growing clones naturally begin to dominate regardless of antibody producing activity.

Cell fusion offers a powerful technique to produce specific antibody to a selected antigen. The proportion of antibody-producing clones is remarkably high and may be due to the fact that spleen cells which are triggered by immunization are particularly successful in giving rise to hybrids (Köhler and Milstein, 1975). The ultimate immunochemical objective of "off the shelf" reagents is brought much nearer by these methods. A variant of the general principle involves injecting hybrid cells into mice to produce solid tumours which may give a serum concentration of $10\,mg\,ml^{-1}$ of antibody to an antigen of interest.

There are obviously problems in these techniques, particularly in terms of hybrid selection and tissue culture technology and, given some luck, the production of hybrid cells making antibody to a macromolecular antigen (i.e. an enzyme or protein) may take 3–4 months. Without luck the procedures may take far longer. The dilemma is, therefore: when should these techniques be attempted rather than conventional immunization and immunoaffinity purification of antibodies to the antigen of interest? The dilemma is highlighted by the fact that classical immunization and antibody preparation need only take 3–4 months.

As usual in immunochemistry a recommendation depends on the antigen of interest and the facilities available to the intended user of the techniques. One consideration is the ease of purification of the antigen of interest and the amount which can be prepared. If sufficient antigen is readily available for an immunization schedule and for the preparation of immunoadsorbent, then the classical approach is perhaps to be recommended. If only very small amounts of antigen are available, and it is prepared with difficulty, then the cell fusion methods are to be recommended, but only when the hybridization and tissue culture technology are conveniently available. Obviously each putative immunochemist must consider all possibilities in trying to reach a decision. However, the Milstein technique provides new and exciting vistas for the immunochemistry of enzymes and proteins.

3
Antiserum Processing

In this chapter methods of antiserum processing and assessment will be described. Although most immunochemical reactions will occur with unfractionated antiserum there are many advantages in using purified immunoglobulins, including reduction in non-specific interactions, e.g. reduction in background staining of immunoprecipitation lines. In general, immunoglobulins should be purified for immunochemical studies and much recent work involves the use of antibodies which are specific for the antigen of interest.

I. Purification of Immunoglobulins

Immunoglobulins are the most basic globulins of the serum. Their solubilities and high isoelectric points relative to other serum proteins form the basis of most purification procedures.

Techniques for serum fractionation include ethanol fractionation, salt fractionation, gel filtration and ion-exchange chromatography. The techniques are described in detail elsewhere (Williams and Chase, 1967; Harboe and Ingild, 1973) but a general procedure for mammalian sera which embodies many suggestions of these authorities (Walker and Mayer, 1977) is described in the Technical Supplement (Chapter 7).

II. Assessment of Antiserum Specificity

It is essential to use several immunodiffusion and immunoelectrophoretic techniques to test the specificity of the antiserum. This is required because the principle and sensitivity of each technique is different and artefacts which suggest multispecificity may occur in some analytical immuno-chemical systems, e.g. with multimeric and membrane protein antigens (Walker *et al.*, 1976). Clearly the assessment of an antiserum is only as good as the sensitivity of the immunochemical analyses. Therefore anti-serum purification should be considered for all antisera even if they appear to be monospecific by the criteria of several immunoprecipitation analyses. For example, an antiserum may be absorbed with a tissue extract which contains a small amount of the antigen of interest, to try to remove contaminating antibodies without great loss of antibodies to the antigen of interest.

The general methods for immunodiffusion and immunoelectrophoretic analyses have been excellently reviewed (Ouchterlony, 1968; Bjerrum and Bøg-Hansen, 1976b), and, therefore only the types of analyses which are particularly suitable for protein antigens will be considered here.

The antiserum should be tested against the crudest tissue preparation available, e.g. detergent-solubilized homogenate. Although this may pro-duce problems of background staining due to non-specific precipitation in immunoprecipitation techniques it precludes the possibility of missing some antigen reaction with antibodies in the antiserum. Most immuno-diffusion and immunoelectrophoretic analyses are conveniently performed in agar or agarose gels.

A. *Immunodiffusion*

Double-diffusion analyses (Ouchterlony, 1968) can be used to identify the number of antigen–antibody systems with a tissue extract and the antiserum (Fig. 2a). These analyses are particularly useful for obtaining reactions of identity, comparing a purified antigen (in one well) with components of an antigen mixture (in a second well) by their reaction with an antiserum (in a third well).

The concentration of the antigens which are in opposition to an antiserum in an immunodiffusion analysis may be varied by serial dilution, e.g. dilutions of a tissue extract around a central antiserum-containing well (Ouchterlony, 1968). Alternatively the amounts of immunoreactants (anti-gens and antibodies) may be varied by opposition of a range of different volumes of tissue extract and antiserum (Piazzi, 1969; Fig. 2b). The advantage of these types of immunodiffusion analyses is that, by varying the amounts of the immunoreactants, latent contaminating antigen–antibody systems may be revealed, e.g. for 6-phospho-gluconate dehyd-rogenase (Fig. 2b). In general the resolution of immunodiffusion analyses is such that they are only suitable for assessment of antisera which contain antibodies to a few macromolecular antigens.

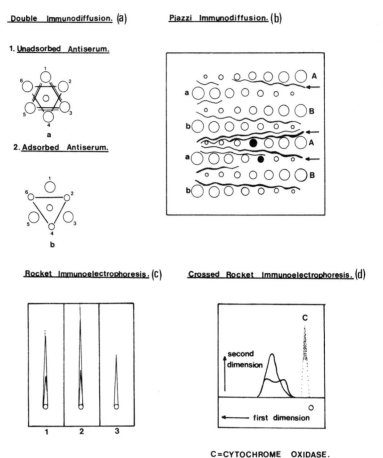

Fig. 2. Immunodiffusion and immunoelectrophoretic analyses. Figs 2a–c show the analyses of antisera before and after adsorption. (a) Wells 1, 3 and 5 contained purified cytochrome oxidase, and wells 2, 4 and 6 contained samples of a particle-free supernatant prepared from homogenate of rat liver. Immunodiffusion was carried out for 2 days at room temperature in a moist atmosphere. (b) Wells contained particle-free supernatant prepared from mammary gland of mid-pregnant (a) and 15 day lactating (b) rabbits. Opposing wells contained unabsorbed antiserum (A) and completely absorbed antiserum (B). The arrowed immunoprecipitate lines did not stain for 6-phosphogluconate dehydrogenase activity. Immunodiffusion was carried out for 24 h at room temperature in a moist atmosphere. (c) Each well contained 10 μl of a particle-free supernatant prepared from mammary glands of 15 day lactating rabbits. Immunoelectrophoresis of the acetyl-CoA carboxylase was carried out for 16 h at 10 V/cm at 15°C with 0·1% (v/v) antiserum in 1% (w/V) agarose gels. Unadsorbed antiserum was present in tracks 1 and 2. Adsorbed antiserum was present in track 3. (d) A mixture of purified cytochrome oxidase and particle-free supernatant proteins were separated by electrophoresis at 20 V/cm for 2 h at 15°C in the first dimension. Immunoelectrophoresis in the second dimension was carried out for 16 h at 10 V/cm at 15°C into a gel containing unadsorbed antiserum (0·25% v/v) to cytochrome oxidase.

It should be noted that multiple immunoprecipitate lines can occasionally be artefacts, e.g. due to refilling wells (Kabat, 1971). Tissue extracts which contain membrane protein antigens may give multiple lines in immunodiffusion analyses. These multiple lines have been interpreted to be the result of differential phospholipid binding to the antigen (Hackenbrock and Hammon, 1975 and Fig. 3b) or to the presence of subunit and holoenzyme in the tissue extract (Poyton and Schatz, 1975). Detergents are usually present in tissue extracts containing membrane protein antigens and can obviously influence the behaviour of the antigens in immunodiffusion analyses. The choice of buffer used for immunodiffusion analysis may be varied to provide conditions which most favour the native state of the antigen. Rabbit antisera give sharp immunoprecipitation lines when the gel buffer contains 0·15 M salt while antisera from fowl give good precipitation lines when the gel buffer contains 0·6 M salt. The addition of protease inhibitors to the gel and sample buffers (e.g. phenylmethane sulphonylfluoride, EDTA or Trasylol) are to be recommended for all forms of immunochemical analysis.

The problems of studies on detergent solubilized membrane proteins in immunodiffusion analyses are shown clearly by work on monoamine oxidase. This enzyme is an integral protein in the outer mitochondrial membrane. Enzymological studies on monoamine oxidase have generated much controversy and interest by indicating that multiple forms of the enzyme may exist as demonstrated electrophoretically (Sandler and Youdim, 1972) and by pharmacological means (Johnston, 1968). The molecular basis for the electrophoretic heterogeneity is likely to be based on differential phospholipid binding (Houslay and Tipton, 1973) to a single gene product (Tipton et al., 1976; Dennick and Mayer, 1977): the molecular basis of the pharmacological heterogeneity may reside in the fact that the enzyme is distributed on both sides of the outer mitochondrial membrane (Russell et al., 1978b). Many authors, most recently Minamuira and Yasunobu (1978), have shown that after detergent solubilization the enzyme fractionates in many analytical procedures into multiple species, particularly molecular weight species. These species are the result of enzyme aggregation in the detergent solution.

It should be clear from this description that monoamine oxidase has all the enzymological and physicochemical properties in detergent solution to be a model of potential immunochemical problems with membrane enzymes. It is no surprise therefore that it does present immunochemical problems (Russell et al., 1978a) which are interesting and from which useful generalities may be noted.

In early immunochemical work with this enzyme (Dennick and Mayer, unpublished observations) it was observed that in immunodiffusion analyses detergent must be present in the gel; otherwise multiple immunoprecipitation lines near to the antigen well were commonly seen. This phenomenon results from the aggregation of the enzyme on entering the detergent-free agarose or agar gel. Recently more detailed immunodiffusion analyses have been carried out with the enzyme in order to try to

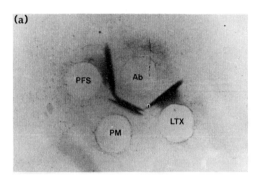

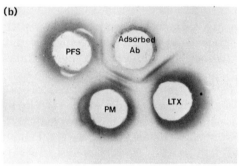

Fig. 3. Immunodiffusion of human liver particle-free supernatant (PFS), purified liver monoamine oxidase (PM) and Triton X-100 extracts of liver mitochondria (LTX) against unadsorbed (a) and adsorbed (b) antiserum to human monoamine oxidase. Immunodiffusion was carried out for 2 days at room temperature in 1% (w/v) agarose in 20 mM potassium phosphate, pH 7·0 containing 0·15 M NaCl and 1.5% (w/v) Triton X-100. Immunoprecipitation lines were stained for protein with Coomassie brilliant blue.

establish the immunochemical relationship of the enzyme in different human tissues (Russell *et al.*, 1978a).

Even with the purified human monoamine oxidase multiple immunoprecipitation lines were generally observed on immunodiffusion: two immunoprecipitation lines (one of which stained for enzyme activity) were seen with freshly prepared enzyme and after storage at −20°C three or four lines were commonly observed (Fig. 3a and b).

Interestingly, although two or more immunoprecipitation lines were given with preparations of the purified enzyme only one line was given with the enzyme in Triton X-100 extracts of liver mitochondria (i.e. the subcellular fraction from which the enzyme was prepared). This indicates that the physiochemical state of the enzyme is different in the two detergent preparations: this state may be dictated by several factors including the protein/detergent ratio and the phospholipid content of the preparation. It is important to note that multiple immunoprecipitation lines are obtained with unadsorbed antiserum (Fig 3a) and with antibodies to monoamine oxidase which have been purified by mitochondrial adsorption (Fig. 3b). Adsorption was performed by binding antibodies to monoamine oxidase onto mitochondria in iso-osmotic conditions followed by elution with 0·2 M glycine-HCl, pH 2·2 and subsequent adjustment to pH 7·0 with 1 M potassium phosphate (Fig. 6).

The fact that multiple lines were obtained with the purified enzyme and not with the enzyme in a detergent extract of mitochondria and that multiple lines (Fig. 3b) were obtained with purified antibodies as well as crude antiserum (Fig. 3a) clearly distinguishes the observed phenomena from those that could be expected if the multiple lines were due to contaminating antigens. These types of phenomena on immunodiffusion or immunoelectrophoresis can clearly complicate interpretation of reactions of identity. Although, as might be expected, multiple lines were obtained on immunodiffusion analysis of detergent-solubilized extracts of human liver, placenta, brain cortex and platelets, clear complete reactions of identity were seen for the enzyme from these different tissue sources (Russell et al., 1978a).

A further problem shown in Fig. 3 is that a subcellular fraction ("particle-free supernatant" prepared by centrifugation of liver post-mitochondrial fraction for 6×10^6 g min), which should not contain mitochondria, does contain immunodetectable monoamine oxidase. This can also be shown by radiochemical assay of enzyme activity (Russell et al., 1978a). This phenomenon may result from detachment of the enzyme from the outer membrane, but this is most unlikely for an integral outer membrane protein. It is much more likely that the "particle-free supernatant" contains microsomal monoamine oxidase, or enzyme attached to outer mitochondrial membrane, or membrane fragments which have sloughed off during homogenization of the tissue.

This observation highlights a major difficulty experienced when examining subcellular fractions immunochemically, namely impurity of the subcellular fractions which may result from artefacts of homogenization or centrifugation. Careful analyses of reactions of identity are called for to distinguish the unexpected presence of an enzyme (or precursor or degradation product) in a subcellular fraction from the possibility of a contaminating antigen–antibody system (Walker *et al.*, 1976).

This type of analysis is vital in biological studies where the site of biosynthesis of proteins or their precursors (e.g. proteins with additional "signal" sequences, Blobel, 1977) is in an organelle distinct from their functional sites, so that some form of translocation mechanism from site of synthesis to functional biological site may occur.

B. Immunoelectrophoresis

In classical immunoelectrophoresis antigens are separated by electrophoresis in one dimension and are then allowed to interact by diffusion with the antiserum in a second dimension (Grabar and Williams, 1953). This provides a much more sensitive means of assessing the specificity of an antiserum than immunodiffusion. Another technique with excellent resolving power for multispecific antisera is cross-over electrophoresis (Moody, 1976), where tissue extract and antiserum are opposed in a gel with the antigen mixture at the cathode and the gel at pH 8·6, such that most antigens but not the antibodies are negatively charged. Electrophoresis forces the antigens towards the antiserum well. Electroendo-osmosis causes the antibodies to move towards the antigens and fine immunoprecipitation lines are rapidly produced (within 40 min).

Electrophoresis of antigens at pH 8·6 into a gel which contains antibodies has been increasingly used in recent years. The antigen may be forced into the antibody-containing gel directly (Fig. 2c, Laurell, 1966) or after electrophoretic separation of the protein mixture at pH 8·6 in the first dimension (Fig. 2d, Weeke, 1973a). Several variations of the latter procedure, including tandem-crossed immunoelectrophoresis (Krøll, 1973a) and crossed line immunoelectrophoresis (Krøll, 1973b), have been developed to add the facility of identification of immunoprecipitation lines to the advantages of resolution and quantitation, which electrophoresis into antibody-containing gels have over classical immunoelectrophoresis.

A whole variety of methods for fractionating antigen mixtures have been used in the first dimension of two dimensional immunoelectrophoresis. Proteins may be separated in the first dimension by means of isoelectric focusing (Söderholm *et al.*, 1975) or electrophoresis in polyacrylamide gels in the presence (Converse and Papermaster, 1975; Webb *et al.*, 1977; Chua and Blomberg, 1979) or in the absence (Loft, 1975; Lundahl and Liljas, 1975; Ekwall *et al.*, 1976) of sodium dodecyl sulphate. As well as providing better antigen resolution these techniques permit the determination of valuable protein parameters such as pI and antigen molecular weight. Problems arising with these methods are that considerable difficulty may be experienced in the correct interfacing the polyacrylamide and agarose gels, and that the subunits of some proteins in sodium dodecyl sulphate may not react with antiserum.

Any antigen fractionation procedure may be immunochemically monitored by means of fused-rocket immunoelectrophoresis (Svedsen, 1973).

Although immunoelectrophoresis into antibody-containing gels gives excellent resolution there are several ways in which artefacts may arise. Multisubunit proteins may dissociate in the low ionic strength buffers used for electrophoresis giving rise to complex immunoprecipitate lines (Paskin and Mayer, 1976). A further complication and one studied in some detail by Bjerrum and Bøg-Hansen (1976b) is the proteolytic modification of antigens and the effect this has on immunoprecipitation lines. Phenomena such as multiple precipitation lines, "split" precipitation lines, "flying" precipitation lines and "skewed" precipitation lines may occur if proteolytic degradation takes place. These effects may result from proteolytic activity in the purified immunoglobulin (e.g. plasmin) or in the tissue extract. Membrane protein antigens are particularly susceptible to proteolysis when extracted from membrane in either ionic or non-ionic detergents and care should be taken to include inhibitors of proteolysis in extraction buffers. For proteins which require the presence of denaturing agents at all times (e.g. keratins) it is possible to perform immunoelectrophoresis in the presence of sodium dodecyl sulphate or urea (Lee et al., 1978).

C. Identification of Antigen–Antibody System of Interest

If an antiserum proves to be multispecific the major problem is to identify the immunoprecipitation line of interest. Only then can the antiserum be purified in order to remove contaminating antibodies.

Enzymes which retain activity in immunoprecipitation lines make identification of the precipitation lines relatively easy assuming that a sufficiently sensitive histochemical stain is available (e.g. dehydrogenases, Fig. 2b or esterases). In this way it is easy to identify the antigen–antibody system of interest (Walker et al., 1976). Alternatively, radioligand binding may be used to identify an immunoprecipitation line of interest (e.g. with radiolabelled neurotransmitter receptor agonists or antagonists; Blomberg and Berzins, 1975; Teichberg et al., 1977).

However, if an enzyme is inactive in an immunoprecipitation line, or the antigen of interest is a catalytically inactive protein, then some other reaction of identity must be employed. Many methods have been designed which rely on the use of purified antigen to identify the immunoprecipitation line which is given by the same antigen, amongst the multiple lines which may be given by a tissue extract. This approach relies on the immunochemical purity of the purified antigen and also requires the availability of purified antigen in sufficient quantities for the analyses. Purified antigens can be used for reactions of identity with the antigen of interest in tissue extract by immunodiffusion (Ouchterlony, 1968) or

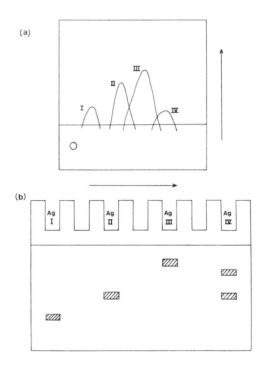

Fig. 4. Determination of antigen subunit molecular weight. (a) A radiolabelled antigen mixture is analysed by crossed-rocket immunoelectrophoresis. (b) The individual immuno-precipitates are analysed by polyacrylamide gel electrophoresis in the presence of sodium dodecyl sulphate. After staining for protein and drying the gel the subunits of each antigen may be identified by autoradiography or fluorography.
Ag = antigen.

immunoelectrophoretic analyses (Axelsen *et al.*, 1973). Monospecific antiserum to some component of interest in an antigen mixture or alternatively a polyspecific antiserum to all components of the mixture except the component of interest can be interposed in an intermediate gel between the antigens resolved by electrophoresis in the first dimension and the multispecific antiserum to be used for second dimensional immuno-

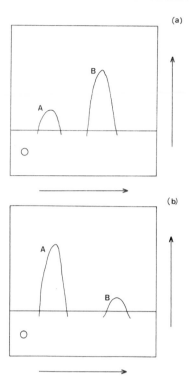

Fig. 5. Analysis of antigen mixtures during antigen purification. The same amount of protein is applied to the sample well from a preparation before (a) and after (b) a step in the purification of antigen A. Antiserum concentration in the gel is the same in both immunoelectrophoresis plates (a and b).

chemical analysis. In this way a component of interest can be positively identifed (Weeke, 1973).

If the subunit molecular weight of an antigen of interest is known, then the gel immunoprecipitate for this antigen may be identified by analysing individual immunoprecipitates, by polyacrylamide gel electrophoresis, in the presence of sodium dodecyl sulphate (Norrild et al., 1977; Walker, unpublished observations). Antigen mixtures labelled radioactively in vivo or in vitro may be analysed by crossed-immunoelectrophoresis, and the individual immunoprecipitates analysed by polyacrylamide gel electrophoresis in the presence of sodium dodecyl sulphate (Fig. 4) followed by autoradiography (Norrild et al., 1977), or fluorography (Walker, unpublished observations). The practical details of these methods are given in the Technical Supplement (Chapter 7).

Alternatively procedures have been used in which antigen mixtures are first resolved by polyacrylamide gel electrophoresis in the presence of sodium dodecyl sulphate and then treated with antiserum. Immunoprecipitates have been subsequently identified by fluorescently labelled second antiserum (Valderrama et al., 1976), by an enzyme-coupled second antiserum (Olden and Yamada, 1977) or with I^{125}-labelled protein A (Burridge, 1978). These methods suffer, however, from the disadvantage that the ability of antibodies to recognize an antigen may be greatly reduced or totally abolished because of the presence of sodium dodecyl sulphate. Any of the two dimensional techniques outlined above may also be used to help identify an antigen of interest when several immunoprecipitates are obtained.

Finally, since the area underneath a rocket immunoprecipitate is proportional to the amount of antigen, crossed-rocket immunoelectrophoresis may be used to monitor antigen purification. The area beneath a rocket divided by the amount of protein in the sample well (at a fixed antiserum concentration) may be used as equivalent to a classical "specific activity" in antigen purification schedules (Fig. 5).

III. Purification of Antibodies to the Antigen of Interest

Antisera can be purified by adsorption procedures (Kwapinski, 1972), in which they are treated with preparations enriched in contaminating antigens. Alternatively, antibodies to the antigen of interest can be purified by use of preparations which are enriched with, or only contain, the antigen of interest (Kabat, 1967).

A. Adsorption of an Antiserum with Contaminating Antigens

Adsorption of an antiserum can be performed with soluble or immobilized contaminating antigens. Antisera to enzymes can be conveniently adsorbed with contaminating antigens in subcellular fractions which contain little or none of the antigen of interest, with contaminating antigens in subcellular fractions prepared from a tissue in a developmental stage at which there is little or no antigen of interest, and with fractions which are discarded during the purification of the antigen of interest (Walker et al., 1976).

The proportion of contaminating antigens required for complete adsorption of an antiserum, can be determined by quantitative immunoprecipitation of the contaminants, quantitative rocket immunoelectrophoresis, the sharpness and intensity of immunoprecipitation lines on immunodiffusion analysis (Walker et al., 1976), or by Sewell titration (Sewell, 1967).

These analyses should be performed when either soluble or immobilized adsorbents are to be used. Adsorption in solution should be performed at equivalence, whereas immobilized contaminants may be used in excess.

Preparations of soluble contaminating antigens can be conveniently used as adsorbents (Walker *et al.*, 1976). Immunoglobulins can be purified from the adsorbed antiserum by techniques described in the Technical Supplement (Chapter 7). This should ensure removal of most of the adventitious proteins in the preparation after adsorption (Mayer, unpublished observations).

Insolubilized contaminating antigens may be used for antiserum adsorption. Contaminating antigens may be insolubilized by polymerization (e.g. with glutaraldehyde). Since gel formation is dependent on protein concentration it is sometimes advisable to add a protein such as bovine serum albumin $(50–100\,mg\,ml^{-1})$ to the dilute preparation of contaminating antigens to ensure rapid gel formation.

When polymerized gels (glutaraldehyde heteropolymers) are used for column chromatography, problems may arise because of the poor flow properties of the material. Adsorption in batches may, therefore, be more convenient. Alternatively contaminating protein antigens may be immobilized onto solid supports (e.g. to Sepharose with cyanogen bromide) for use in adsorption procedures.

Sepharose-immunoadsorbents, prepared by coupling proteins from a subcellular fraction enriched with a contaminating antigen, are very conveniently used. These immunoadsorbents have good flow properties or alternatively can be easily used in batches.

Naturally there are problems with immunoadsorbents prepared by polymerization of proteins, or coupling proteins to solid supports. Polymerization or immobilization of antigens may reduce their antigenicity and this should be estimated and allowed for when determining the quantity of an adsorbent to be used. Another problem is related to the use of protein preparations enriched with contaminating antigens which also invariably contain some of the antigen of interest. This means that the concentration of antibodies to the antigen of interest will be depleted by the immunoadsorption procedures. However, loss of some antibodies to the antigen of interest is a small price to pay for removal of all the contaminating antibodies.

The production of tissue-specific antisera is a relatively easy process. A polyspecific antiserum (e.g. multi-tissue antiserum) may be conveniently mixed with glutaraldehyde heteropolymers or acetone powders derived from tissues other than the one of interest. Antisera specific for different developmental stages in the life span of an organism may be prepared in an analogous manner.

B. Adsorption of an Antiserum with Antigen of Interest

Although appealing in principle, the binding of antibodies to some preparation of the purified antigen and its subsequent elution present some problems particularly for the enzymologist. Several procedures have been developed whereby purified antigen is bound to a solid support (Chapter 4). The immunoadsorbent is then used to bind specific antibodies which can subsequently be eluted. For example fibrinogen and ovalbumin have been coupled to Sepharose (Bouma and Fuller, 1975) and then used to purify their respective antibodies. Alternatively antibodies can be bound to polymerized antigen (e.g. casein, Houdebine and Gaye, 1976).

From these examples it is apparent that these techniques are often used for proteins which can be obtained in relatively large amounts so that enough antigen is available to adsorb a significant volume of antiserum. However, antisera to enzymes have been purified in this way. Antiserum to fatty acid synthetase has been purified with Sepharose-fatty acid synthetase (5 mg fatty acid synthetase, Alberts et al., 1975). Reutilization of immunoadsorbents increases the usefulness of small quantities of immobilized antigen.

The main problem with the use of immobilized antigen of interest as immunoadsorbent is the quality of the antigen. If a purified antigen is immunologically impure (Chapter 2), and the same antigen is used to prepare the immunoadsorbent, then contaminating antibodies could be bound to the immobilized antigen. The situation is complex and depends on the degree of purity of the antigen and the relative immunogenicities of the antigen of interest and the contaminants. Finally, binding of antibodies (or antigens, Chapter 4) to immunoadsorbents is complicated by non-specific binding of proteins, e.g. non-specific immunoglobulins. This necessitates the use of washing procedures to try and elute these proteins before elution of the antibodies of interest, e.g. with 0·15 M NaCl or 0·1 M NaHCO$_3$ (Alberts et al., 1975) or with detergent–salt mixtures (Smith et al., 1978).

Convenient partial adsorption procedures (i.e. not with purified antigen of interest) for membrane antigens can be carried out if the membrane fraction can be easily isolated. Antibodies to monoamine oxidase have been partially purified by adsorption to mitochondrial preparations and elution by low pH. The method is shown in detail in Fig. 6. By this procedure approximately 4% of the protein in the IgG fraction bound to the mitochondrial preparation. The eluted antibodies to monoamine oxidase retained approximately 60% of the immunoinhibitory capacity of the unadsorbed IgG fraction.

IgG (containing antibodies to the enzyme) is mixed with a mitochondrial preparation (in 100 mм-sodium phosphate buffer, pH 7·2 in the proportion of 2 mg of IgG protein to 1 mg of mitochondrial protein. Suspension incubated at 4°C for 2–3 h.

↓

Centrifuge for $10^5 g_{av.}$ min. Pellet is washed twice with 20 mм-sodium phosphate buffer containing 0/15 м NaCl.

↓

Washed pellet incubated with 0·2 м glycine-HCl, pH 2·8 volume equal to the original volume of the IgG preparation) for 1 h at 0°C with constant stirring.

↓

Centrifuge for $225 \times 10^3 g_{av.}$ min. Supernatent is immediately neutralized with 1 м potassium phosphate, pH 7·2.

↓

Solution dialysed overnight at room temperature against 20 mм sodium phosphate, pH 7·0 containing 0/15 м NaCl.

Fig. 6. Partial purification of antibodies to monoamine oxidase by mitochondrial adsorption.

Elution of antibodies of interest can be achieved with a variety of agents. The aim of these treatments is to break the electrostatic and hydrophobic interactions which bind antigens to antibodies. Low pH (e.g. 0·2 м glycine-HCl, pH 2·6), high pH (e.g. 1 м ammonium hydroxide, pH 11·5), high salt concentration (e.g. 4·5 м $MgCl_2$) and chaotrophic salts (e.g. 3 м NaSCN) and м propionic and acetic acids have been used to release antibodies (or antigens) from immunoadsorbents.

Comparison of several eluants for the removal of casein antibodies from a Sepharose-casein immunoadsorbent have been carried out (Al-Sarraj, White and Mayer, unpublished observations). The effects of 2·5 м sodium iodide, pH 9·0 and 3 м sodium thiocyanate, pH 6·8 were compared with 0·2 м glycine HCl, pH 2·8. The sodium iodide and sodium thiocyanate were removed from the antibody preparations by Sephadex G-25 chromatography and the glycine-HCl was rapidly neutralized with 1 м Tris solution. In all cases the preparation of eluted antibodies was cloudy and centrifugation of each suspension resulted in sedimented protein. The ratio of supernatant protein concentrations in the centrifuged eluants was approximately 4:2:1 for glycine-HCl, thiocyanate and iodide respectively. It is probable that the combination of differential elution and differential denaturation resulted in the different concentrations of eluted antibodies. The effectiveness of the antibody preparations in immunoprecipitating casein is shown in Fig. 7. There is a marked reduction in the capacity of each preparation of purified antibodies to immunoprecipitate casein.

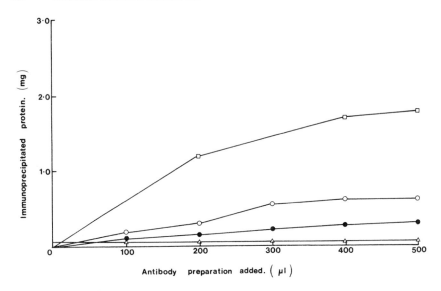

Fig. 7. Immunoprecipitation of casein by adsorbed antibody preparations. Antibody preparations were prepared by eluting samples of Sepharose-casein immunoadsorbent with 0·2 M-glycine HCl, pH 2·8 (○); 2·5 M sodium iodide, pH 9·0 (●); and 3 M sodium thiocyanate, pH 6·8 (△). Antibody preparations were processed as described in the text. Antibodies in unadsorbed antiserum (IgG) are shown for comparison (□). Casein (6 μg) was added to each sample, the volume adjusted to 1 ml with phosphate-buffered saline and immunoprecipitation was allowed to proceed for 4 days at 4°C.

Antibodies eluted with glycine-HCl maximally precipitate about 30% of the casein immunoprecipitated by unadsorbed antiserum. This contrasts with the 60% of immunoinhibitory capacity shown by the monoamine oxidase antibody preparation which was eluted from a mitochondrial preparation by glycine-HCl. The ratio of maximally immunoprecipitated caesin was 4:2:⅔ with antibody preparations eluted with glycine-HCl, thiocyanate and iodide respectively, which is in very good agreement with the ratio of protein concentrations in these antibody preparations (see above).

It is highly probable (although not proven by this experiment) that denaturation of eluted antibodies results in antibody precipitation. As shown in Fig. 7, the immunoprecipitative capacity of the antibody preparations is a function of their antibody concentrations. Again the individuality of each antigen–antibody system and immunoadsorption method is illustrated (cf. antibodies to casein and monoamine oxidase) in terms of the effect of eluants on immunochemical behaviour of the eluted antibodies. It is clear that much more work on the selection of elution solvents and conditions is required in order to prepare antibodies in maximum yield.

Attempts have been made to separate antigen–antibody complexes by milder procedures including ion exchange chromatography (McCauley and Racker, 1973) and electrophoresis (Dean *et al.*, 1977). The affinities of the eluted antibodies must be considered, namely whether all the antibodies are eluted in the described conditions or whether the eluted antibodies are those with weaker affinities for the macromolecular antigen. The latter situation could be advantageous if the eluted antibodies were to be used to prepare an antigen binding immunoadsorbent. It should be possible to elute antigen from such an immunoadsorbent under carefully defined conditions.

Antibody subpopulations responding to different antigenic determinants can be purified by techniques including immunoadsorption (Arnon, 1973; McCans *et al.*, 1975) and in the same way antibodies to catalytic and non-catalytic sites on enzymes or different oligomeric forms of proteins (Pages *et al.*, 1976), may be fractionated by immunoadsorption procedures.

In spite of the technical problems purified antibodies to an antigen of interest are of great value in immunochemical studies (Chapter 5) especially since they considerably reduce non-specific phenomena in immunoprecipitation and immunoaffinity procedures.

Purified antibodies are much easier to use and give much clearer results in immunoprecipitation reactions in gels. Problems of background staining are avoided and this means that the quantitative measurements (e.g. rocket immunoelectrophoresis, Mancini Immunodiffusion) can be made more easily. Furthermore, if immunoprecipitation or immunoadsorption (immunoaffinity) techniques are to be used to immunoisolate antigens from tissue extracts, purified antibodies avoid many of the problems of non-specific precipitation and non-specific adsorption respectively, which can plague these techniques when unpurified IgG is used.

Criticisms of adsorption of antisera with immunoadsorbents prepared with the antigen of interest (i.e. based on antigen quality, see above) may be overcome if adsorption with preparations enriched with contaminating antigens precedes adsorption with antigen of interest. In this way antibodies to contaminating antigens could be removed first and would, therefore, not bind to those contaminating antigens which may contaminate the antigen of interest which has been used to prepare the immunoadsorbent.

IV. Reassessment of Antiserum Specificity

The success of adsorption procedures with either contaminating antigens

(a)   (b)

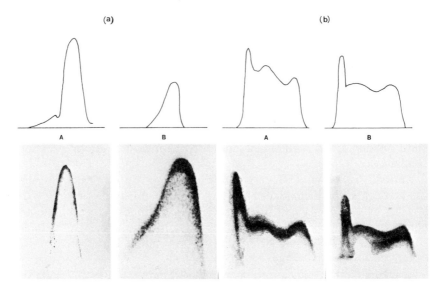

Fig. 8. Crossed-rocket immunoelectrophoresis of ^{32}P-labelled recombined casein and ^{32}P-labelled tissue extract from mammary gland of lactating rabbit. Immunoelectrophoresis was carried out in 1% (w/v) agarose gels. The ^{32}P-labelled preparations were prepared as described by Al-Sarraj *et al.* (1978). Coomassie Blue staining of the gels of ^{32}P-labelled recombined casein (a) and ^{32}P-labelled tissue extract (b) tested against unadsorbed antiserum (A) and adsorbed antiserum (B). Radioautograms of each crossed-rocket are shown beneath their respective Coomassie stained rockets.

or the antigen of interest must be assessed qualitatively and quantitatively. The techniques for assessment are those described previously, and the procedures are used to test for the monospecificity of the antiserum (Fig. 2).

Cross-rocket immunoelectrophoresis is a very sensitive technique to observe the effects of adsorption on the specificity of an antiserum qualitatively. Even in a case where an antiserum is very specific before adsorption (i.e. casein, Al-Sarraj *et al.*, 1978) cross-rocket immunoelectrophoresis can be used to provide evidence for minimal qualitative alteration in antibody specificity, during antibody purification from the IgG fraction (Fig. 8) by immunoaffinity chromatography.

Simple Ouchterlony double diffusion is often adequate to demonstrate the complete removal of contaminating antibodies by immunoadsorption. Immunodiffusion is best when a small number of antigen–antibody systems are known to be detectable by a multispecific antiserum. Clear demonstration of the removal of contaminating antibodies by adsorption of a multispecific antiserum to cytochrome oxidase with a fraction enriched in contaminating antigens is shown in Fig. 9 (Walker *et al.*, 1976).

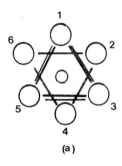
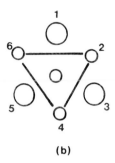

Fig. 9. Ouchterlony double diffusion analysis with unadsorbed and adsorbed antiserum. Diffusion was performed in 1% (w/v) agarose gels containing 20 mM sodium phosphate buffer, pH 7·0, 150 mM sodium chloride and 1% (w/v) Triton X-100. Wells 1, and 5 contained purified enzyme, and wells 2, 4 and 6 contained samples of a particle-free supernatant prepared from homogenate of rat liver. The central wells contained (a) unadsorbed antiserum; (b) completely adsorbed antiserum by cytochrome oxidase. Immunodiffusion was carried out for 2 days at room temperature in a moist atmosphere.

Since the purification techniques may result in some loss of antibody titre the relative titre of the adsorbed antiserum should be estimated, e.g. by rocket immunoelectrophoresis (Fig. 2c, d).

Alternatively quantitative immunoprecipitation may be used to assess loss of antibodies during an adsorption procedure. An example of this method is shown for casein antibodies in Fig. 7.

4

Uses of Antisera

In this section the uses of antisera which are of value to cell and molecular biologists, enzymologists and protein chemists will be discussed. Antisera may be used to determine the amounts of protein antigens and their rates of synthesis and degradation. Antisera may also be used to identify protein antigens in different subcellular compartments, in different cells or occasionally in different species. Antisera are routinely used to isolate and purify protein antigens from tissue extracts.

Antisera are very convenient surface probes: they can be used to localize protein antigens by a variety of techniques, including immunohistochemical techniques. The vectorial orientation of enzymes in membranes can also be conveniently established with antisera. Immunoinhibition of catalytic activity can be measured to establish if an active site of an enzyme is oriented externally or internally on a cell surface membrane (i.e. plasma membrane) or organelle membrane (e.g. mitochondria and microsomes).

I. Determination of Antigen Amount

Methods for the estimation of the amount of a protein antigen include quantitative precipitation of an antigen from solution, quantitative immunoprecipitation in gels, measurements which are dependent on immunotitration of enzyme activity, radioimmune assays and more recently enzyme-immune assays.

Quantitative precipitation was developed by Heidelberger and Kendall (1929) and is based on the observation that the addition of increasing amounts of a soluble antigen to a series of tubes containing a constant volume of antiserum results initially in an increase in the amount of precipitate formed until a maximum is reached. At equivalence of antigen and antibody an estimate can be obtained of the antibody content of the serum expressed in terms of added antigen.

A standard curve which relates amount of precipitate to the amount of antigen in the presence of excess antibodies can be produced. The amount of antigen in a preparation can, therefore, be measured. However, methods for measuring the amount of precipitated protein are not very sensitive and other procedures have been designed to estimate the amount of an antigen. These procedures will be described and compared in terms of their relative value to biological scientists.

A. Quantitative Immunoprecipitation in Gels

Agar or agarose gels are frequently used as support media in which antigens and antibodies may react and the most valuable techniques are those in which antibodies are incorporated into the support medium (e.g. into 1% w/v agarose in an appropriate buffer system). Antigen amount can be estimated by single radial immunodiffusion (Mancini et al., 1965) where antigen diffuses into an antibody containing gel. Initially antigen concentration around the antigen well is high so that the antigen diffuses away from the well and forms soluble immune complexes until the concentration of antigen falls to a value at which immunoprecipitation occurs. This gives rise to an immunoprecipitation ring around the well. The area of this ring gives a measure of the amount of antigen in the preparation which is being tested. Naturally this technique can be used with a monospecific antiserum but if residual enzyme activity can be used to mark the immunoprecipitation ring then a multispecific antiserum can be used. In this case the single immunodiffusion analysis is carried out with a tissue extract or biological fluid and the immunoprecipitation line of interest is identified by means of a histochemical stain for enzyme activity. Multispecific antisera have been frequently used in this way, e.g. by geneticists to estimate the amount of a gene product in extracts from a number of genetically different organisms (Lanzerotti and Gullino, 1972).

An alternative method of estimating antigen amount is rocket immunoelectrophoresis. The principle of immunoprecipitation is similar to that described for single radial immunodiffusion, except that the antigen is forced into the antibody containing gel by electrophoresis. In this case an immunoprecipitation "rocket" is produced, the height (or area) of which is proportional to the amount of antigen in the sample of the tissue extract. Histochemical techniques can also be used with this method where appropriate.

Immunoprecipitation lines of interest can also be visualized by radioligand binding and autoradiography, e.g. binding of radioactive bungarotoxin to immunoprecipitated postsynaptic cholinergic receptor (Teichberg *et al.*, 1977).

Rocket immunoelectrophoresis can be a very sensitive and convenient technique to estimate the amount of an antigen. Sensitivity will naturally depend on the specific antigen–antibody system under study, but 1–5 µg ml^{-1} of antigens in tissue extracts or biological fluids can be readily estimated. The amount of casein in mammary explants at different times after hormonal stimulation (Al-Sarraj *et al.*, 1979) can be conveniently measured by this technique. Immunoelectrophoresis was carried out as described by Axelsen *et al.* (1973). Agarose gel (1% w/v) containing

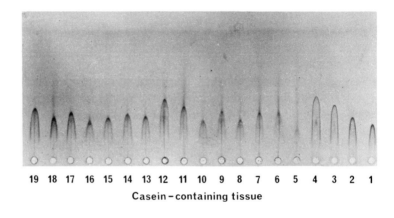

19 18 17 16 15 14 13 12 11 10 9 8 7 6 5 4 3 2 1

Casein – containing tissue

Fig. 10. Quantitative determination of casein by means of rocket immunoelectrophoresis. Wells 1–4 contained 18, 36, 54 and 72 ng of rabbit recombined casein polypeptides as standards. The other wells contained particle-free supernatant (2–10 µl) from freshly prepared explants (well 5); from explants cultured for 24, 48, 72 and 96 h with hormones (insulin, prolactin and cortisol; wells 6, 12, 17 and 19); from explants cultured after the removal of hormones for 24 h (wells 7, 8 9 and 10) or 48 h (wells 13, 14, 15 and 16) and from explants cultured throughout in the absence of hormones (wells 11 and 18). Electrophoresis was carried out as described by Weeke (1973b) at 0·5 V cm^{-1} for 16 h at approximately 15°C.

adsorbed antiserum (76 µg protein ml^{-1} of gel; Al-Sarraj *et al.*, 1978) was used. Adsorbed antiserum is recommended since it eliminates background staining when gels are stained with Coomassie Blue after electrophoresis. This increases the accuracy of measurement of peak area (or height) which is proportional to the amount of antigen in each sample. Purified antigen (i.e. recombined casein polypeptides) was used as standard (Fig. 10). Often "flying rockets", i.e. not dropping to the sample well, are obtained; the reasons for this are not understood. Nevertheless measurement of rocket height from the centre of the sample well gives a good measure of antigen amount. A linear relationship between rocket height and amount

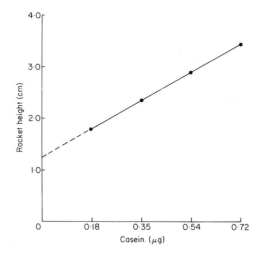

Fig. 11. Standard curve relating rocket height to amount of antigen. The validity of this method of antigen quantitation can be conveniently verified by an alternative technique, e.g. Mancini Radial Immunodiffusion.

of casein is obtained (Fig. 11). The reason for the line not passing through the origin is again not understood but is often found in rocket immunoelectrophoresis (Weeke, 1973b).

B. Measurements Coupled to Enzyme Activity

The interaction between enzymes and their respective antibodies generally leads to a reduction in enzyme activity (Arnon, 1973). The enzyme may be completely inhibited, partially inhibited or in exceptional cases enzyme activity is stimulated. A correlation has been found between substrate size and the extent of immunoinhibition, i.e. greater inhibition is achieved with larger substrates (Cinader and Lafferty, 1964). Often stimulation occurs only when enzyme activity is assayed with poor substrates or when mutant enzymes with poor catalytic activity are studied.

Immunotitration of enzyme activity is commonly used as a measure of the amount of an enzyme in a tissue extract or biological fluid. The titrations are based on the assumption that the volume of antiserum required to completely immunoinhibit enzyme activity is proportional to the amount of the enzyme in the tissue extract or biological fluid. The specific activity of an enzyme (e.g. activity per unit protein or per unit DNA) may change after some physiological stimulus as a result of activation or inactivation, or because the concentration (i.e. number of

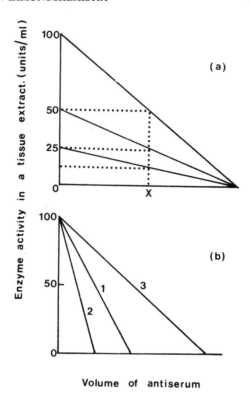

Fig. 12. Immunotitration of enzyme activity. (a) Titration of the same amount of an enzyme of different specific activities. Volume of antiserum (X) required for 50% inhibition of enzyme activity. (b) Titration of activated or inactivated enzyme in a tissue extract relative to enzyme activity before change. Activity before change (1); two-fold activation of enzyme (2); two-fold inhibition of enzyme (3).

enzyme molecules) has either increased or decreased. This distinction is fundamental to the acute (changing activity of pre-existing enzyme) and chronic (changing the number of enzyme molecules) regulation of metabolic pathways. Demonstration of changing activity or amount of an enzyme is of paramount importance to the interpretation of all experiments in which enzyme activity is measured in biological systems in non-steady state conditions.

Two alternative immunochemical approaches have been used. In one approach increasing volumes of antiserum are added to fixed volumes of tissue extract (obtained from a living organism in a defined physiological state) in separate incubation tubes, and the volume of antiserum (or the extrapolated volume) required for complete inhibition of enzyme activity is used as a measure of enzyme-antibody equivalence (Fig. 12). Alternatively increasing enzyme activities from a tissue extract are added to a fixed volume of antiserum and the extrapolated point at which enzyme activity can first be measured is taken as a measure of the equivalence of antigen and antibody (Figs 14 and 15). In the first approach equal enzyme activities from tissues in different physiological states should require the same volume (or extrapolated volume) of antiserum for complete inhibition when enzyme amount is changing. In the second approach equal enzyme activities from tissue extracts should be inhibited to exactly the same extent when enzyme amount is changing.

Both approaches have been successfully used to distinguish enzyme amount changes for activity changes and are therefore described.

Immunochemical measurements of enzyme amount have been carried out by determination of the volume of antiserum which is required to completely inhibit the enzyme activity. A common method is to mix increasing volumes of antiserum with fixed volumes of tissue extract. Each mixture is usually incubated at 30–37°C for some time, e.g. 30 min (not if the enzyme is heat-labile) and then incubated at 4°C for a prolonged period (e.g. overnight). This technique has been varied so that incubations were carried out for much shorter periods (e.g. Peavy and Hansen, 1975). Each incubation mixture is then centrifuged to remove immunoprecipitated enzyme and enzyme activity in the supernatant assayed. Alternatively enzyme activity has been measured in preparations which have not been centrifuged where the rapid anti-catalytic effect of antibodies is seen (Hizi and Yagil, 1974). The volume of antiserum required for complete inhibition of enzyme activity must often be an extrapolated volume, or alternatively the volume required for 50% inhibition of enzyme activity can be measured. This is necessary even when measurements are made on supernatants prepared by centrifugation of suspensions to remove immunoprecipitates, which may contain residual enzyme activity (Betts and Mayer, 1977). This may be explained by the relative activities of free enzyme and enzyme–antibody complexes in conditions of equivalence or antibody excess.

The measurement of enzyme amount is based on the existence of a linear relationship between the amount of an enzyme and the volume of antiserum required to completely immunoinhibit enzyme activity. This assumes that changes in specific activity of an enzyme for any reason are not associated with loss of a significant number of antigenic determinants (Fig. 12a).

Immunotitration of an enzyme can be used to examine the nature of the change in enzyme activity in a cell after some physiological stimulus. It is possible to distinguish if an enzyme has been activated or inactivated or if its amount has changed. If the change in enzyme activity is due to activation or inactivation of a pre-existing amount of enzyme then im-munotitration of enzyme activity would be as shown in Fig. 12b. If the amount of the enzyme changes as a consequence of the stimulus then immunotitration of the same number of units of enzyme activity in tissue extracts before and after the stimulus should require the same volume of antiserum for complete inactivation. In such cases the volume of antiserum

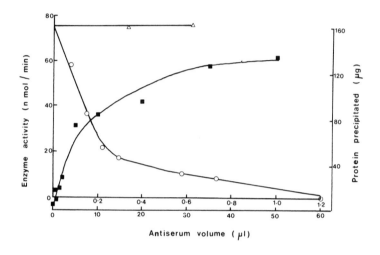

Fig. 13. Immunoinhibition of an enzyme which is independent of immunoprecipitation. Immunotitration of acetyl-CoA carboxylase with monospecific antiserum. Enzyme activity after treatment with control serum ($\triangle$), and antiserum ($\bigcirc$). Immunoprecipitated protein ($\blacksquare$).

required for complete inhibition of enzyme activity can be used as a measure of the amount of the enzyme in the tissue (e.g. Betts and Mayer, 1977).

There are some complications in the use of these procedures. However, two considerations deserve mention here. Firstly the volume of antiserum required to completely inhibit enzyme activity is that required to quantita-tively precipitate the enzyme. It is advisable to measure enzyme activity in supernatants after centrifugation to remove immunoprecipitates if prob-lems of interpretation of immunotitrations are to be avoided as in studies on glucose 6-phosphate dehydrogenase in mouse (Hizi and Yagil, 1974) and rat liver (Peavy and Hansen, 1975). However, in some cases im-munoinhibition of enzyme activity is not linked to precipitation of the enzyme (e.g. Fig. 13, Manning and Mayer, unpublished observations). Here enzyme activity is completely inhibited by the addition of a very small volume of antiserum relative to that required to precipitate the enzyme. This phenomenon may be due to depolymerization of the highly polymerized form of the enzyme which is required for the activity of acetyl-CoA carboxylase (Walker *et al.*, 1976). This type of phenomenon may occur quite frequently.

Secondly, as previously noted, it is usual for incomplete inhibition of enzyme activity to occur on adding increasing volume of antiserum to a fixed enzyme activity. This means that a residual enzyme activity can be measured irrespective of how much antiserum is added. To avoid this problem calculation of the volume of antiserum for 50% inhibition of activity can be carried out (see above). However, for better accuracy the addition of increasing enzyme activities to a fixed volume of antiserum is often preferred because it minimizes the extrapolative errors used in calculating antigen–antibody equivalence.

Immunotitration of pyruvate dehydrogenase and fatty acid synthetase in rat adipose tissue in the perinatal period is shown in Figs 14 and 15. Clearly in all cases an identical equivalence point is obtained which shows that the change in the activity of pyruvate dehydrogenase (3–5 fold) and fatty acid synthetase (20–60 fold) in the perinatal period is caused by a fall in the amounts of the enzymes in the tissue. This is a very important observation which could not be obtained without immunochemical methods. Further studies are now in progress to characterize the molecular basis (i.e. changed enzyme synthetic or degradative rates) by which these changes are brought about (Sinnett-Smith, Vernon and Mayer, unpublished observations).

Several points of immunochemical interest arise from these studies. Short incubation periods were used for both antigen–antibody interactions. This is necessary since both enzymes are inactivated considerably on remaining at 4°C for any length of time. Obviously a compromise is necessary between loss of enzyme activity in tissue extracts and the time required for immunoinhibition of enzyme activity. Preliminary experiments were therefore carried out to find the minimal time required for maximal immunoinhibition in antiserum excess. This experiment leads to the choice of times indicated in Figs 14 and 15. This type of preliminary experiment is necessary for all immunoenzymological studies with unstable enzymes.

Two points of general interest arise from these studies. Firstly the immunotitrations were carried out with crude sera, i.e. prepared by taking the supernatant from clotted blood. Immunotitration is probably the only immunochemical technique where such a preparation could be recommended. Secondly, the immunotitrations were carried out with xenogeneic antisera. The antiserum to pyruvate dehydrogenase was raised in sheep against the enzyme from pig heart, and the antiserum to fatty acid synthetase was raised in sheep against the enzyme from rabbit mammary gland. The use of xenogeneic antisera is a matter of empirical observation.

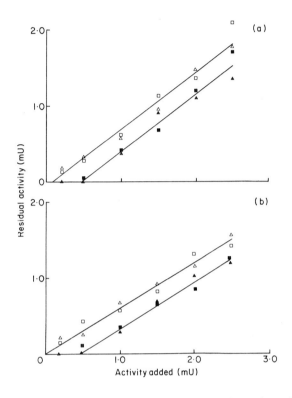

Fig. 14. Immunotitration of pyruvate dehydrogenase from rat adipose tissue. Incubation of fixed volumes of antiserum with increasing enzyme activity were carried out for 15 min at 4°C. Incubation mixtures were centrifuged for 6 min at 14 000 g_{av} before assay. Total pyruvate dehydrogenase was assayed by the method of Stansbie *et al.* (1976). Each symbol represents the mean of six measurements at 2 days *prepartum* and three measurements at 2 days *post partum*. Lines were determined by linear regression analyses. Immunotitration of pyruvate dehydrogenase from (a) parametrial, (b) subcutaneous adipose tissue. Animals killed at 2 (■) days *prepartum* and 2 (▲) days *post partum*. Titration with control sera are shown by open symbols (□, △).

Sometimes antisera cross-react very well with antigens from other species, but they sometimes fail to react at all (e.g. anti-rabbit casein does not react with human or rat casein). Finally, it should be noted that the non-specific effects of control serum and antiserum on the activity of fatty acid synthetase should be the same, i.e. the lines in Figs 15a and b should be parallel. The reason for their divergence is probably due to the fact that the products of the fatty acid synthetase reaction, long chain fatty acids, inhibit the enzyme reaction. However, serum albumin binds fatty acids and therefore prevents this inhibition. The protein concentration of the control

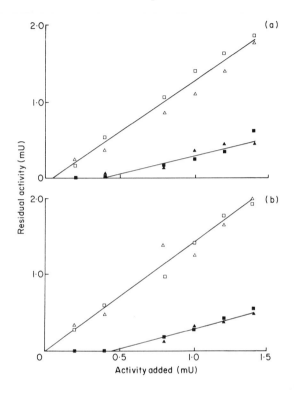

Fig. 15. Immunotitration of fatty acid synthetase from rat adipose tissue. Incubations of fixed volume of antiserum with increasing enzyme activity were carried out for 2 h at 4°C. Incubation mixtures were centrifuged for 6 min at 14 000 $g_{av.}$ before assay. Fatty acid synthetase was assayed by the method of Speake *et al.* (1975). Experimental conditions, expression of results and symbols are the same as those described in Fig. 14.

serum was twice that of the antiserum and, therefore, more inhibition of enzyme activity should occur in the latter case. Even activation of the enzyme may occur in the presence of control serum due to binding of fatty acids to serum albumin and possibly other proteins. Activation or inhibition of enzymes by serum components may be a common occurrence in immunotitration studies. This type of problem may be overcome by the use of purified specific antibodies.

C. Radioimmune and Enzyme-immune Assays

Radioimmune assays (Fig. 16) which employ the principle of competitive binding of antibodies to radio-iodinated antigen and to antigen in biological fluids have been used for many years (Hunter, 1967). Such systems are currently used for the assay of many peptide hormones (Collins and Hennam, 1976) and for protein (Bolton and Hunter, 1973) and enzyme (Roberts and Painter, 1977) antigens.

Radioimmune assays for proteins or enzymes are extremely sensitive and specific but need to offer a good working range over which the amount of antigen can be measured. Iodinated antigens are extensively used in radioimmune assays. However, iodination of proteins may cause modification of their molecular properties (Krohn *et al.*, 1977) which could affect any of the parameters needed for a good radioimmune assay of a protein. Indeed the highest specific radioactivities of a radioiodinated protein may only be achieved with considerable antigen modification (Hunter, 1967). The use of lactoperoxidase catalysed iodination may cause less antigen modification, in that it labels predominantly tyrosine residues in certain proteins (Krohn *et al.*, 1977). Iodination of proteins certainly alters their antigenic properties when measured by immunoadsorbent techniques (Mayer and Walker, unpublished observations).

A major consideration in the design and use of a radioimmune assay for proteins is the availability of a method for separating free protein antigen from antigen–antibody complexes, since this is fundamental for competitive binding assays. Separations by electrophoresis, ion-exchange chromatography, gel filtration and solvent and salt precipitation have been used. Several authors have used double antibody techniques where an antiserum to the IgG fraction which contains the antibodies of interest (e.g. rabbit antiserum to sheep IgG) may be used to precipitate the antibody–antigen complexes of interest (Hunter, 1967).

More recently techniques for the isolation of antibody–antigen complexes by binding to *Staphylococcus aureus* (containing protein A, Jonsson and Kronvall, 1974; see Chapter 7, Section X) or by precipitation with polyethylene glycol (Creighton *et al.*, 1973) have been developed. Naturally a procedure must be specifically designed for the antigen and antiserum of interest, since there are so many differences in the molecular and physicochemical properties of protein antigens.

Two interesting and potentially extremely useful developments are the immunoradiometric (Miles and Hales, 1968a, b; Readhead *et al.*, 1973; Woodhead *et al.*, 1974) and two-site assays (Catt and Tregear, 1967; Addison and Hales, 1971; Ling and Overby, 1972). These differ from

Ag and Ab = antigen and antibody

Long period

1. nAg + $nAg^{125}I$ + nAb $\longrightarrow$ $\frac{n}{2}Ag + \frac{n}{2}Ag^{125}I + Ab\frac{n}{2}Ag + Ab\frac{n}{2}Ag^{125}I$

   unknown   labelled   limiting
   (e.g. Ag =   antigen   amount
   $Ag^{125}I$)   (e.g. $\frac{1}{2}[Ag +$
                      $Ag^{125}I])$

(Simplified to assume high affinity antibody and one combining site per antibody molecule)

2. $\frac{n}{2}Ag + \frac{n}{2}Ag^{125}I + Ab\frac{n}{2}Ag + Ab\frac{n}{2}Ag^{125}I \longrightarrow \underbrace{\frac{n}{2}Ag + \frac{n}{2}Ag^{125}I}_{\substack{\text{measure} \\ \text{radioactivity} \\ \text{(free)}}} + \underbrace{Ab\frac{n}{2}Ag + Ab\frac{n}{2}Ag^{125}I}_{\substack{\text{measure} \\ \text{radioactivity} \\ \text{(bound)}}}$

separate
bound and
free species

3. Plot bound/free versus known antigen concentration to obtain standard curve so that unknown antigen concentration can be estimated.

Fig. 16. Radioimmunoassays.

classical radioimmune assays in that antibodies instead of antigen are iodinated and immonoadsorbents are used to great advantage.

The immunoradiometric assay is shown in Fig. 17. The technique was developed for polypeptide hormones. The advantages of the method over radioimmune assay are that all the unknown antigen reacts with antibodies at least once and the immunocomplex product is assayed against a low background. Furthermore, since the antigen is not modified by iodination, little interference in the reaction of the antigen with the specific antibodies should occur. The sensitivity of the technique is substantially increased since specific antibodies are attached to an immunoaffinity matrix before iodination. In this way at least one antigen binding site on each antibody molecule is protected during the iodination procedure, i.e. the site which is interacting with antigen. The other site may or may not be damaged by the procedure. The iodinated reagent is usually eluted from the immunoadsorbent with low pH. Low avidity antibodies are first removed by washing with dilute HCl at pH 3 and the required high avidity antibodies are then eluted with dilute HCl at pH 2. The assay depends on the selection of iodinated antibodies with very high affinity for antigen so that very low concentrations of antigen in biological fluids can be detected. The most satisfactory storage procedure for iodinated antibodies (up to two months) has been found to be recombination of the antibodies with the immunoadsorbent and storage at −20°C. Antibodies are then eluted as described previously when needed for assay.

Non-specific protein effects are minimized if standards are prepared in the biological fluid containing the antigen (e.g. serum). The principle of the assay is similar to a radioimmune assay in that it involves an initial prolonged incubation (e.g. up to five days) and subsequent separation of immunocomplex from unreacted reagent (in the case of immunoradiometric assays this is iodinated antibody). This is nicely achieved again with an immunoadsorbent to the antibodies of interest. Shortly after mixing a large excess of immunoadsorbent with the assay mixture (e.g. 30 min) the antibody-immunoadsorbent complex is removed by centrifugation and the supernatant radioactivity (which is proportional to the amount of antigen in the biological fluid) is measured.

There is no reason to think that the technique should be less effective with enzymes and proteins than it is with polypeptides. The disadvantage of the technique is centred on the recurrent problem of a requirement for a relatively large amount of antigen for the preparation of immunoadsorbents. For many proteins there would be no problem in this respect but many tedious enzyme purification schemes result in very small quantities (e.g. 0·5–1·0 mg) of purified enzyme, most of which may be consumed in an immunization schedule. However, methods of this type, where anti-

A. *Preparation of Reagent*

1. Matrix + Ag $\xrightarrow{\begin{array}{c}\text{coupling procedure}\\ \text{(e.g. coupling Ag to}\\ \text{diazotized amino cellulose)}\end{array}}$ Immunoadsorbent
   (e.g. cellulose)   (M-Ag)

2. M – Ag + antiserum $\longrightarrow$ M – Ag – Ab_{sp}
   where Ab_{sp} = specific antibodies

3. M – Ag – Ab_{sp} + ^{125}I $\longrightarrow$ M – Ag – $Ab_{sp}^{125}I$

B. *Assay*

1. M – Ag – $Ab_{sp}^{125}I$ $\xrightarrow[\text{(e.g. by low pH)}]{\text{Dissociation}}$ M – Ag + $Ab_{sp}^{125}I$

2. Ag + $Ab_{sp}^{125}I$ $\longrightarrow$ $(Ag - Ab_{sp}^{125}I)$ + $Ab_{sp}^{125}I$
   (unknown) (excess) (long period at 4°C)

3. $(Ag - Ab_{sp}^{125}I) + Ab_{sp}^{125}I + M - Ag \longrightarrow M - Ag - Ab_{sp}^{125}I + (Ag - Ab_{sp}^{125}I)$
   (short period at 4°C)

4. M – Ag – $Ab_{sp}^{125}I$ + $(Ag - Ab_{sp}^{125}I)$ $\xrightarrow{\text{centrifuge}}$ Supernatant $(Ag - Ab_{sp}^{125}I)$
                                                                    (measure radioactivity)
   (to pellet the M–Ag–$Ab_{sp}^{125}I$)

Fig. 17. Immunoradiometric assay procedure.

bodies are iodinated, will clearly avoid problems associated with iodinated protein (e.g. decreasing immunogenicity, difficulties in iodinating protein antigens, problems caused by the presence of detergents in membrane protein preparations).

An alternative assay of antigen amount which needs less antiserum and may offer potential increases in assay sensitivity, precision and specificity is the two-site assay procedure (Fig. 18). The method involves the coupling

A. *Preparation of Reagent*

1. Matrix + Ab ────────▶ Immunoadsorbent reagent
   (e.g. cellulose paper $(M - Ab_{sp})$
   or polypropylene or
   polyethylene centrifuge
   tubes)

B. *Assay*

$$\text{incubate}$$

1. $M - Ab_{sp} + Ag$ ────────▶ $M - Ab_{sp} - Ag$
   Ab excess'   unknown (e.g. 24 h at 4°C)

2. $M - Ab_{sp} - Ag + Ab_{sp}{}^{125}I$ ────────▶ $M - Ab_{sp} - Ag - Ab_{sp}{}^{125}I$
   (e.g. 24 h at 4°C)

3. Remove immunoadsorbent from tube or preferably wash tubes carefully and measure radioactivity.

Fig. 18. Two-site assay procedure.

of unlabelled antibody to an insoluble matrix (e.g. cellulose or surfaces of plastic tubes) which can then be used as a means of extracting antigen from biological fluids. The major proviso of the method is that the antigen should have more than one immunological group (determinant) so that its uptake on to the immunoadsorbent can be measured by the subsequent reaction of a second labelled antibody.

The amount of antigen needed to make the immunoadsorbent which is used to purify the specific antibodies may be reduced, since the antibodies adsorbed on to the centrifuge tubes or matrix need not be as pure as the labelled antibody used in the assay. However, this may increase non-specific binding problems. Therefore, specific antibodies bound to the support matrix and for use as labelled reagents are probably preferable.

The advantages of the technique are increased sensitivity resulting from the immunological extraction of the antigen from the biological fluid, low non-specific radioactivity and the fact that when antibodies are immobilized on tubes no separation stage of the assay is necessary. Disadvantages are centred on the fact that repeated washings are required necessitating the use of antibodies with very low antigen–antibody dissociation constants.

The two-site method probably offers the most potential for enzymologists and protein chemists for the reasons previously mentioned, particularly since antigen modification is not required and great sensitivity may be ensured by the multiple antigenic determinants which are often present on the surface of protein macromolecular antigens. Certainly two-site assays in plastic centrifuge tubes would offer the greatest advantage of all to busy biological scientists.

Radioimmune assays have also been developed (Bolton and Hunter, 1973) which use immobilized antibodies (e.g. coupled to Sepharose). Naturally methods based on this type of immunoadsorbent again preclude the need to devise separation techniques although non-specific binding to the immunoadsorbent may affect the sensitivity and specificity of the methods.

Enzyme-immune assays based on the use of immobilized antigens or antibodies have also been developed (Hamaguchi *et al.*, 1976 a,b; Papermaster *et al.*, 1976). The principle of the use of immobilized antigen is described below. Antigen is coupled to Sepharose by a cyanogen bromide procedure. The assay involves two stages. In the first stage competitive binding of antibodies to immobilized antigen and to free antigen in the biological fluid occurs. As the amount of free antigen in the biological fluid increases, less antibodies bind to the immobilized antigen. In the second stage of the assay antibody binding to the immobilized antigen is estimated with a second antiserum to the IgG containing antibodies to the antigen of interest. This second antiserum is modified by covalently linking the immunoglobulins to an enzyme which has easily measurable activity (e.g. alkaline phosphatase). The proportion of enzyme activity which is immobilized is, therefore, an indirect and amplified measure of the amount of antigen in the biological fluid. The sensitivity of assays for the enzyme can be optimized with fluorogenic substrates (e.g. methylumbelliferone phosphate).

Recently enzyme-immune assays have been developed with reagents attached to glass rods (Hamaguchi *et al.*, 1976b). The principle of the method is outlined in Fig. 19. The binding of the F_{ab}-β-D-galactosidase complex is proportional to the amount of antigen. Therefore the quantity of the 4-methylumbelliferone produced by the galactosidase is proportional to the amount of antigen. The use of glass rod immunoadsorbents decreases problems of non-specific binding of the F_{ab}-β-D-galactosidase complex compared to particulate matrices (e.g. Sepharose) and improves reproducibility considerably by decreasing the handling problems encountered with particulate reagents. The specificity and sensitivity of the immunoadsorbents could possibly be significantly improved by the use of purified antibodies (i.e. purified by immunoaffinity chromatography) for the preparation of the glass rod absorbents. Reasons for the development

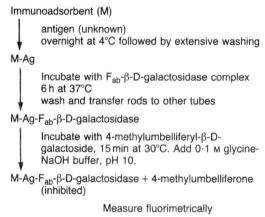

This method uses glass rods as solid phase.

A. *Preparation of Immunoadsorbent*

Pyrex glass rods (5 × 3 mm)

↓ coat with 3-aminopropyl triethoxysilane

Aminoalkylsilyl glass

↓ 1% glutaraldehyde

"Activated" glass

↓ IgG from antiserum of interest followed by extensive washing

Immunoadsorbent

B. *Preparation of Antibody-Fab- -D-galactosidase complex*

The complex is prepared by coupling F_{ab} fragment and β-D-galactosidase with N_1N^1-O-phenylenedimaleimide

C. Assay

Immunoadsorbent (M)

↓ antigen (unknown) overnight at 4°C followed by extensive washing

M-Ag

↓ Incubate with F_{ab}-β-D-galactosidase complex 6 h at 37°C wash and transfer rods to other tubes

M-Ag-F_{ab}-β-D-galactosidase

↓ Incubate with 4-methylumbelliferyl-β-D-galactoside, 15 min at 30°C. Add 0·1 M glycine-NaOH buffer, pH 10.

M-Ag-F_{ab}-β-D-galactosidase + 4-methylumbelliferone (inhibited)

Measure fluorimetrically

Fig. 19. An enzyme-immune assay.

of enzyme-immune assays include cost relative to radioimmune assays, danger associated with radioimmune assays, and the short half-life of radioactive isotopes of iodine.

D. Radioimmune Assays of Small Molecules: Cyclic Nucleotides

Many radioimmune assays for small molecules have been developed and used to great advantage in clinical situations (e.g. for steroids, prostaglandins and many drugs). Biological scientists increasingly want to assay very small quantities of metabolites. These metabolites may be very unstable or subject to rapid alteration of concentration following some physiological stimulus. Immunochemical methods theoretically offer a very specific

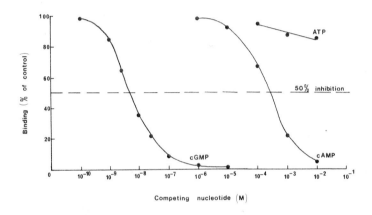

Fig. 20. Binding of [³H]-cGMP to antibodies in the presence of unlabelled cGMP, cAMP or ATP. [³H]-cGMP (2 nM) was incubated with antiserum (final dilution 1/40) and known concentrations of competing nucleotides in 50 mM Tris HCl buffer, pH 7·5 containing disodium EDTA (4 mM) in a final volume of 200 μl for 2 h in an ice/water bath. Bound [³H]-cyclic GMP was determined by precipitation with ammonium sulphate followed by centrifugation.

system for the rapid isolation and quantitation of these substances. Much interest has been shown in the last few years in determining the concentrations of cyclic nucleotides in cells in different physiological states. Assaying the concentration of these substances is difficult, involving radioactive prelabelling of nucleotide pools or use of preparations of specific binding proteins. Antibodies to cyclic nucleotides provide ideal "specific binding proteins". Production of antisera to these molecules involves rendering them haptenic by coupling to some large macromolecule (i.e. protein). Radioimmune assays are subsequently carried out by competitive binding techniques.

Very specific antisera to cyclic GMP have been produced and used in this manner (e.g. Steiner, 1974; Strange and Dymond, unpublished observations, described below). Cyclic GMP is succinylated at the 2^1-O-position (Cailla *et al.*, 1976) and subsequently conjugated with human serum albumin (Steiner, 1974). Several rabbits are immunized with a total of 0·25 mg of the succinyl-cGMP-albumin complex emulsified in Freunds complete adjuvant by injection at two subcutaneous (shoulders) and two intramuscular sites (hind legs). Each animal further receives a set of four injections at fortnightly intervals for two months and then at monthly intervals. The immune response of the animals varies somewhat but after ten weeks of immunization high titres of specific antibodies were obtained. For example, after this time specific antibodies were given with high affinity for cGMP and low cross-reactivities with cAMP, ATP, GTP, GDP, 5'-GMP, cCMP, cIMP and cUMP. Such an antiserum was used in a radioimmune assay of cGMP (Fig. 20); the assay was developed in order to measure the concentration of cGMP in mouse neuroblastoma cells after treatment with various agonists. The measurement of cGMP concentration was in very good agreement with measurements made using a [^{3}H]-guanine prelabelling method for measurement of cGMP (Strange, 1978). This specific example illustrates the potential of immunochemical methods for the measurement of the concentrations of cellular metabolites.

E. General Conclusions

The biological scientist must decide on one or more of the methods to measure the amount of a protein antigen. The choice will ultimately be tailored to the specific antigen of interest where consideration should be given to the molecular and physicochemical properties of the protein and the nature of the tissue extract or biological fluid to be used.

The amounts of antigens in tissue extracts vary considerably so that the same antigen can be present in biological fluids or tissue extracts at markedly different concentrations. The method of quantitation used will vary according to the concentration of antigen present. For example, the amount of α-foetoprotein may be estimated in foetal plasma or amniotic fluid ($10^{-6} - 10^{-1}$ g ml^{-1}) by immunodiffusion or immunoelectrophoretic methods but estimated in normal plasma ($10^{-9} - 10^{-8}$ g ml^{-1}) only by radio immune assay (Leek and Chard, 1974). Enzymes ($10^{-6} - 10^{-4}$ g ml^{-1}) can be measured by immunodiffusion or immunoelectrophoretic methods (e.g. acetyl-CoA carboxylase; Manning *et al.*, 1976; Walker *et al.*, 1976). The sensitivity of immunoassays which are coupled to enzyme activity depends on the molecular activity of the enzyme and sensitivity of the assay method (e.g. radiochemical assays are often most sensitive) and allow $10^{-7} - 10^{-6}$ g ml^{-1} of enzyme to be measured. Immunoassays linked to enzyme activity, immunodiffusion and immunoelectrophoresis are limited by the volume of biological fluid or tissue extract which can be used for the estimations, e.g. 5–20 µl for immunoelectrophoresis and immunodiffusion depending on well-size, 10–500 µl for assays linked to enzyme activity depending on the nature of the assay (e.g. spectrophotometric or radiochemical) and reactant concentration (e.g. affecting specific radioactivity of substrate). These practical limitations probably mean that these methods are less sensitive (e.g. 1–2 orders or magnitude) than radioimmune or enzyme-immune assays where $10^{-10} - 10^{-8}$ g ml^{-1} of antigen can usually be estimated (Leek and Chard, 1974; Hamaguchi et al., 1976).

II. Reactions of Identity

Antisera have been used in phylogenetic studies where the existence of conformation homology has been corroborated by immunological cross-reaction (Arnon, 1971). The nature of antigenic determinants on macromolecules has been examined by conformational alteration of proteins (Arnon, 1971) or by inspection of the immunological relationships of peptide fragments obtained from proteins (Arnon, 1971; Beeley, 1976). The uses of reactions of identity are illustrated in several sections of this book, particularly in Chapter 3.

There are cases where controversy exists with regard to the number of enzymes which mediate a given reaction in a tissue. For example, multiple substrate specificities and differential pharmacological susceptibilities have been described for monoamine oxidase, and the possibility exists that there are at least two forms of the enzyme. Whether these forms are different gene products is contentious. Antiserum the enzyme, was found to immunoprecipitate the enzyme and concurrently inhibit oxidation of substrates specific for both forms of the enzyme, and a substrate common to the two putative forms of the enzyme (Dennick and Mayer, 1977). The volume of antiserum required to immunoprecipitate all of the enzyme was also that required to completely inhibit each of the substrate activities. This type of data, although sometimes equivocal, can be used with reactions of identity, to decide if multiple gene products are present in particular cell types.

III. Immunoisolation Procedures

Immunoisolation procedures are very useful for cell and molecular biologists, enzymologists and protein chemists. For example, enzymologists frequently wish to study the acute or chronic regulation of enzyme activity in tissues. Rapid (acute) changes in enzyme activity may be mediated by some covalent modification of a protein (e.g. phosphorylation). Slower (chronic) changes in enzyme activity are mediated by changes in the amount of an enzyme in a tissue. Changes in the amount of an enzyme can be achieved by altering its rate of synthesis or degradation in response to a stimulus. Measurement of covalent enzyme modification or rates of enzyme synthesis or degradation requires isolation of the enzyme from a tissue extract. For all these measurements it is best to isolate an enzyme rapidly in order to avoid possible modification of the enzyme in a laborious purification procedure. Antibodies provide a rapid way to isolate an enzyme from a tissue extract. The specificity of antibodies is fundamental to their use and is possibly only equalled by some affinity chromatography systems (Don and Masters, 1975).

All these developments rely on the quality of techniques for the immunoisolation of antigens. Two alternative procedures, immunoprecipitation and immunoadsorption (immunoaffinity chromatography) are extensively used. A method of immunoisolation involving *S. aureus* as adsorbent is also described in Chapter 7, Section X.

A. Immunoprecipitation Methods

In these methods it is usual to add carrier enzyme or protein to a radiolabelled tissue extract or biological fluid. Subsequently enough monospecific antiserum is added to give an excess over antigen (1–2 fold) and the mixture is incubated in conditions to immunoprecipitate the enzyme. Incubation conditions vary but often consist of a short period (e.g. 30 min) at 30–37°C followed by prolonged (overnight or much longer) incubation at 4°C to ensure complete immunoprecipitation (Maurer, 1971). Immunoprecipitates can be removed by centrifugation (e.g. 80 000 × g min), washed repeatedly with iso-osmotic saline and analysed for incorporated radioactivity.

Carrier enzyme is often required to ensure a reasonably sized precipitate. This may represent a significant limitation of the method. The amount of carrier enzyme needed for each immunoprecipitation varies considerably depending on the required size of the precipitate but may be between 5–50 μg. In most experiments many samples need to be analysed (e.g. 10–20) and therefore, since often small amounts of purified carrier enzyme are available (e.g. 1–5 mg), a restriction is set on the possible number of immunoprecipitations which can be carried out. Partially purified enzyme could be used as carrier but this may aggravate problems of coprecipitation (see below).

Careful controls are essential for immunoprecipitation analyses. Two basic problems are non-specific precipitation and coprecipitation. Non-specific precipitation is due to non-specific interactions between the proteins in a tissue extract and immunoglobulins. Also, proteins may simply adhere to the walls of incubation or centrifuge tubes in the absence of control serum. These interactions can be measured with control serum. Control serum is added to tissue extrasts and the incubations processed exactly as described for antiserum. In this way the contribution of non-specifically precipitating material to an immunoprecipitate can be estimated.

Coprecipitation is a significant problem of immunoprecipitation analysis. Adventitious protein is often trapped in immunoprecipitates as they are formed. The degree of contamination of immunoprecipitate depends on the amount of carrier added and therefore the size of the immunoprecipitate. At least three approaches have been taken to overcome this problem: control treatments have been devised to correct for coprecipitation; methods have been designed to minimize coprecipitation; and techniques have been developed for further analysis of immunoprecipitates.

Two methods for the estimation of coprecipitation have been developed. Schimke *et al.* (1965) have designed a control based on two immunoprecipitations from the same tissue extract. Carrier enzyme is first added to the extract, followed by antiserum and immunoprecipitation occurs. After removal of the precipitate the same amount of carrier enzyme is added to the extract and a second immunoprecipitation carried out. The principle of the method assumes that all of the antigen of interest and accompanying coprecipitants will be in the first immunoprecipitate while only the coprecipitants will be in the second immunoprecipitate. Subtraction of radioactivity precipitated in the second case from that precipitated in the first case should give the radioactivity incorporated into the antigen.

A second method for the assessment of coprecipitation has been developed by Cho-Chung and Pitot (1968). Carrier (a) is added to a radiolabelled tissue extract and twice the amount of carrier (b) is added to another equal volume of the same tissue extract. If no coprecipitation occurs then the radioactivity precipitated should be identical in both cases. If coprecipitation occurs then radioactivity incorporated into the antigen of interest is given by

$$A - (B - A)$$
where A = radioactivity in precipitate a
B = radioactivity in precipitate b
since $B - A$ = coprecipitated radioactivity.

Attempts have been made by several authors to minimize the extent of coprecipitation. Since coprecipitation occurs by non-specific trapping similar coprecipitants should be precipitated with immunoprecipitates to any antigen. This has led to the development of pre-immunoprecipitation techniques. Tissue extracts are treated with appropriate quantities of an antigen and antiserum (e.g. ovalbumin-anti-ovalbumin serum) before treatment with carrier enzyme and antiserum to the antigen of interest.

A study of the effects of pre-immunoprecipitation on the subsequent immunoprecipitation of 6-phosphogluconate dehydrogenase from mammary gland illustrates some of the problems and results which may be obtained with this approach (Betts and Mayer, unpublished observations). Enzyme was radiolabelled *in vivo* with L-[4,5-^{3}H]-leucine and immunoprecipitates prepared from a 6×10^6 g min supernatent of mammary gland homogenate. The extent of coprecipitation with this antigen–antibody system, i.e. d.p.m. not in the enzyme subunits (after polyacrylamide gel electrophoresis in the presence of sodium dodecyl sulphate) as a percentage of total immunoprecipitated radioactivity is approximately 25% (Fig. 21a). This is small coprecipitation compared to that seen in some other systems where radioactivity coprecipitated can exceed radioactivity in antigen of interest.

The antigen chosen for the preliminary immunoprecipitation from the radiolabelled supernatant fraction was yeast alcohol dehydrogenase to which an antiserum was available in the laboratory. Although a choice of convenience this antigen–antibody system illustrates several immunochemical points of interest. The analysis of the alcohol dehydrogenase immunoprecipitate by polyacrylamide gel electrophoresis in the presence of sodium dodecyl sulphate (Fig. 21b) revealed several radioactive bands. Immunoprecipitation of alcohol dehydrogenase was accompanied by the loss of approximately 15% of 6-phosphogluconate dehydrogenase activity and, interestingly, a band migrating approximately in the same place as the subunit of 6-phosphogluconate dehydrogenase (Fig. 21b, arrow) contained approximately 15% of the radioactivity in the subunits of the enzyme. The reason for this observation is not completely clear and may be due either to some specific immunoprecipitation of the 6-phosphogluconate dehydrogenase by the antiserum to yeast alcohol dehydrogenase or to the mammary enzyme being a coprecipitant of the yeast antigen–antibody system. If the former explanation is correct then the chance selection of the yeast alcohol dehydrogenase antiserum may be useful in that it points to some evolutionary preservation of antigenic features of yeast and animal dehydrogenases.

While possibly useful for that purpose the pre-immunoprecipitation technique was not successful in reducing the extent of co-precipitation when the tissue extract was subsequently treated with antiserum to

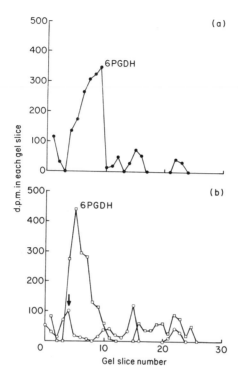

Fig. 21. Analysis of immunoprecipitates by electrophoresis on polyacrylamide gels in the presence of sodium dodecyl sulphate. L-[4, 5-³H]-leucine (1 mCi) was injected *in vivo* into a duct of the mammary gland of a 2 day *post partum* rabbit. After 4–6 h, the gland was excised and a particle-free supernatant prepared ($6 \times 10^6 \, g_{av.}$ min). (a) Immunoprecipitation of 6-phosphogluconate dehydrogenase (6 PGDH) from samples (200 µl) of this supernatant was carried out with the addition of 20 µg of partially purified enzyme as carrier. Incubation was carried out for 30 min at 30°C and overnight at 4°C. To ensure complete precipitation of the enzyme, the volume of antiserum used was twice that required to precipitate all the enzyme present. (b) Yeast alcohol dehydrogenase (25 µg) and its antiserum (200 µl) were added to a sample (200 µl) of particle-free supernatant for preliminary immunoprecipitation. The sample was incubated for 30 min at 37°C and 30 min at 4°C. Subsequently 6-phosphogluconate dehydrogenase was immunoprecipitated as described above. After incubation, the immuno-precipitates were sedimented by centrifugation and boiled in electrophoresis sample buffer for two minutes. After electrophoresis, the gels were cut into 2 mm slices, digested with hydrogen peroxide and radioactivity measured. Electrophoresis of immunoprecipitate of 6-phosphogluconate dehydrogenase (●), alcohol dehydrogenase (○) and 6-phosphogluconate dehydrogenase after preliminary immunoprecipitation (□).

6-phosphogluconate dehydrogenase. The extent of coprecipitation was the same as in the absence of pre-immunoprecipitation (i.e. approximately 25%; Fig. 21b).

The results show that pre-immunoprecipitation was of no use in improving the subsequent immunoprecipitation of the antigen of interest.

Naturally generalizations cannot be made from this since as usual each antigen–antibody system must be considered on its own merits. The main problem with this approach is that coprecipitants may vary for different antigen–antibody systems and, more importantly, that they are present in

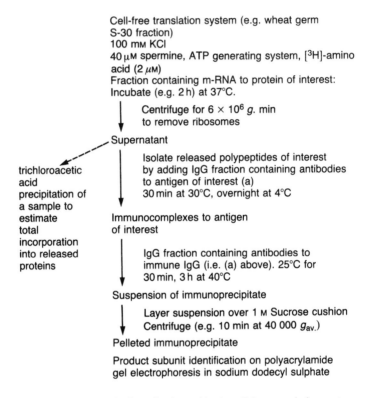

Cell-free translation system (e.g. wheat germ S-30 fraction)
100 mM KCl
40 μM spermine, ATP generating system, [^{3}H]-amino acid (2 μM)
Fraction containing m-RNA to protein of interest: Incubate (e.g. 2 h) at 37°C.

↓ Centrifuge for 6 × 10^6 g. min to remove ribosomes

Supernatant

trichloroacetic acid precipitation of a sample to estimate total incorporation into released proteins

Isolate released polypeptides of interest by adding IgG fraction containing antibodies to antigen of interest (a) 30 min at 30°C, overnight at 4°C

Immunocomplexes to antigen of interest

↓ IgG fraction containing antibodies to immune IgG (i.e. (a) above). 25°C for 30 min, 3 h at 40°C

Suspension of immunoprecipitate

↓ Layer suspension over 1 M Sucrose cushion Centrifuge (e.g. 10 min at 40 000 g$_{av.}$)

Pelleted immunoprecipitate

Product subunit identification on polyacrylamide gel electrophoresis in sodium dodecyl sulphate

Fig. 22. Immunoprecipitation of polypeptides in cell-free translation systems.

such quantities that they cannot be removed by simple preliminary immunoprecipitation techniques.

Other attempts to reduce coprecipitation include washing immunoprecipitates with detergents (Hopgood et al., 1973) and centrifuging immunoprecipitates through a 1 M-sucrose cushion (cf. Figs 22 and 23). It is hoped that co-precipitants may be removed from the immunoprecipitates by this procedure (Rhoads et al., 1973).

Although some success has been achieved by all of these techniques there is room for improvement. Perhaps the use of purified antibodies (Chapter 3), rather than purified immunoglobulins and the use of partially purified extracts may reduce some of these problems.

The best way of assessing coprecipitation is by analysing immunoprecipitates by polyacrylamide gel electrophoresis in the presence of sodium dodecyl sulphate (e.g. Hopgood *et al.*, 1973). This approach should be used in conjunction with a technique designed to reduce coprecipitation.

The technique depends on the immunoreactivity of polysome-bound nascent polypeptide chains of the antigen of interest. A typical procedure is shown below.

Polysomes

(e.g. in 50 mM Tris-HCl buffer, pH 7·5 containing
150 mM NaCl, 5 mM MgCl₂, 1 mg/ml heparin)

    ↓   incubate with IgG from non-immunized animal to
           reduce non-specific binding of antibodies to
           ribosomes

Treated Polysomes

    ↓   Add detergent (e.g. Triton X-100; final concentration
           0·5% w/v). Add appropriate amount of antibodies
           (purified by immunoadsorbent chromatography)
           Incubate 20–30 min.

Antibody-Polysome Complex

    ↓   Add IgG fraction containing antibodies to
           antibodies of interest. Incubate 60 min.
           Centrifuge 10 min at 40 000 g_{av}.

Immunoprecipitated Polysomes

    ↓   Resuspend in starting buffer, layer on 1 M
           sucrose cushion. Centrifuge 10 min at
           40 000 g_{av}.
           Repeat 3–4 times

Immunoprecipitated Polysomes

    ↓   Specific m-RNA extraction in phenol-sodium
           dodecyl sulphate

Specific m-RNA to enzyme or protein
of interest

Fig. 23. Immunochemical isolation of polysomes translating m-RNA of interest.

This procedure will allow the measurement of radioactivity incorporated into the subunit(s) of an enzyme or protein and can clearly identify subunits of coprecipitants. Therefore radioactivity incorporated into the antigen of interest can be measured. It is advisable to compare the radioactivity profile from precipitates obtained with control serum and antiserum and even to analyse precipitates given with different amounts of carrier antigen. The method will not distinguish radioactivity in subunits of equal size derived from different proteins.

Another problem which can be encountered with immunoprecipitation is low incorporation of radioactivity into an antigen, e.g. by pulse-radiolabelled amino acid *in vivo* into a slowly synthesized protein. Furthermore the antigen may be multisubunit (e.g. cytochrome oxidase with 7–8 subunits). In these conditions low radioactivity in the separated peptides may be expected. The immunoprecipitate may often be predominantly immunoglubulin (e.g. possibly 90% immunoglobulin in immunoprecipitates of cytochrome oxidase; Walker and Mayer, unpublished observations). These problems mean that the radioactivity in any band on a polyacrylamide gel may be so low as to be undetectable. In such cases another technique for immunoisolation of an antigen (i.e. immunoadsorption) must be used in order that only antigen and not predominantly immunoglobulin can be loaded on a polyacrylamide gel.

Several methods based on immunoprecipitation have been successfully used to isolate antigens from a wide range of tissue extracts and for a variety of purposes. The variety of these approaches shows the extreme usefulness of immunochemical techniques to biological scientists.

Antisera have been used to isolate newly synthesized polypeptides from *in vitro* protein translation systems (Fig. 22; Rosen *et al.*, 1975) and to isolate polysomes by reaction of antibodies with polysome-bound nascent polypeptide chains (Fig. 23; Palacios *et al.*, 1972). The latter method together with the finding that poly(A) is present in most mRNAs has greatly facilitated the isolation and characterization of mRNAs coding for specific proteins and allows the synthesis of complementary DNA (Houdebine, 1976; Houdebine and Gaye, 1976). Both these procedures (Figs 22 and 23) rely on a double antibody technique to immunoprecipitate the antigen of interest and centrifugation of the immunoprecipitate through a sucrose cushion to remove contaminating proteins.

Studies on rapid covalent enzyme modification such as may occur *in vivo* during acute regulation of some metabolic pathway can be very effectively carried out immunochemically. For example an antiserum to acetyl-CoA carboxylase from rabbit mammary gland (raised in sheep) has been used to rapidly immunoisolate the enzyme from fat cells prepared from rat epididymal fat-pads. The antiserum was used to precipitate the enzyme from cell-homogenate supernatants (prepared by centrifugation for $100\,000\,g_{av.}$ for 60 minutes or $10\,000\,g_{av.}$ for 1 min). The antiserum was only incubated with the cell extracts for 30 min at 30°C (which leads to a 90% loss of enzyme activity) and the immunocomplexes were sedimented by centrifugation at $80\,000\,g$ for 30 min. Over 80% of purified [^{14}C]-biotin-labelled enzyme which was added to such supernatants could be sedimented by these procedures. The short incubation of antibodies with tissue extract followed by rapid sedimentation of immune complexes by high speed centrifugation is of obvious value to those interested in acute enzyme regulation by covalent modification (e.g. by phosphorylation or glycosylation) since the enzyme of interest can rapidly be isolated with minimal alteration of the modified protein. This is a prerequisite when examining physiological change in the extent of covalent modification.

The extent of phosphorylation of acetyl-CoA carboxylase in fat cells has been examined by the method described above. The results are shown in Fig. 24. Clearly the phosphorylated enzyme is immunoprecipitated by

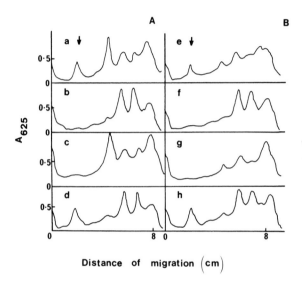

Distance of migration (cm)

Fig. 24. Densitometric traces of radioautographs demonstrating the specific precipitation of ^{32}P-labelled protein from a $10\,000\,g$ supernatant of fat cells after incubation with antiserum to acetyl-CoA carboxylase. Fat-cells were incubated for 75 min with ^{32}P$_i$ with (A) or without (B) insulin (10 m-i.u./ml) added for the last 15 min. After centrifugation of the whole-cell extracts at $10\,000\,g$ for 1 min, the supernatants were incubated for 30 min at 30°C with either antiserum to acetyl-CoA carboxylase (c, d, g and h) or control serum (a, b, e and f) (20 μl/ml in each case). Samples were then centrifuged at $80\,000\,g$ for 30 min at 4°C and the proteins from the supernatant (a,c,e and g) and pellet (b,d,f and h) fractions separated on adjacent tracks by SDS/polyacrylamide-slab-gel electrophoresis (5% gel). The dye front (Bromophenol Blue) was allowed to migrate 10 cm. The arrow indicates the position of the subunit of acetyl-CoA carboxylase.

antiserum and not by control serum. The other peaks in the sedimented material are due primarily to phosphorylated proteins of particulate origin (e.g. pyruvate dehydrogenase).

As an alternative to rapid sedimentation of immune complexes by centrifugation (total isolation time approximately 1 h) is immunoadsorbent chromatography (see below). For example an immunoadsorbent to pyruvate dehydrogenase completely binds the enzyme from rat liver in 15 min at room temperature (Fig. 28; Burgess, Russell and Mayer, unpublished observations) while an immunoadsorbent to fatty acid synthetase from mammary gland binds the enzyme in extracts of mammary tissue within 5 min (Paskin and Mayer, unpublished observations). With some development immunoaffinity chromatography can be carried out much quicker than the time required to prepare cell extracts, which therefore becomes limiting in this type of study.

One specific and advantageous use of immunoprecipitation is for studies on glycoproteins.

Immunoprecipitation techniques coupled with polyacrylamide gel electrophoresis in the presence of sodium dodecyl sulphate can be used to considerable advantage when the antigen of interest is a glycoprotein. The heavy subunit of immunoglobulin can serve as internal standard for carbohydrate identification since it is glycosylated. Therefore carbohydrate staining (i.e. with Periodic-acid-Schiffs reagent) or carbohydrate labelling with lectins (i.e. I^{125} or fluorescein labelled lectins) can be carried out with some confidence (Cahill and Morris 1979). Iodinated protein A, which binds to the F_c portion of immunoglobulins can also be used effectively (Burridge, 1978).

B. Immunoadsorption Methods

Immunoaffinity (Immunoadsorption) techniques may prove the ultimate methods of choice with antibodies. A considerable number of approaches have been taken, some of which are described below.

Several immunoadsorption methods have been developed for the isolation of antibodies (Chapter 3) or antigens with immobilized immunoadsorbents (Kristiansen, 1976). Immunoadsorbents may be prepared in several ways including direct polymerization (Ternynck and Avrameas, 1976) and coupling of antigens or antibodies to insoluble supports e.g. Sepharose, polyacrylamide (Ternynck and Avrameas, 1976) or nylon (Edelman and Rutishauser, 1974). Immunoglobulins from non-immune sera should be coupled to Sepharose for use in control experiments. The immunoadsorbents can be conveniently packed into Pasteur pipettes, syringe barrels, small glass columns, or may be used in batches. Clearly the binding and elution conditions for each antigen–antibody system must be studied. The use of protein A bearing *Staphylococcus aureus* as immunoadsorbent is described in detail in the Technical Supplement (Chapter 7, Section X).

Purified immunoglobulin has been routinely linked to Sepharose (Fig.

24) by cyanogen bromide procedures (Porath *et al.*, 1973) and to polyacrylamide or nylon by bifunctional reagents, e.g. glutaraldehyde (Edelman and Rutishauser, 1974; Ternynck and Avrameas, 1976). Practical details of these procedures are given in the Technical Supplement (Chapter 7).

In general the coupling of relatively high concentrations of antibodies is preferred if the immunoadsorbent is to be used to isolate an antigen from a tissue extract. However, coupling of increasing amounts of antibodies may result in a progressive increase in the number of inactivated antibodies due to factors including unfavourable orientation of the antibodies on the solid support (Kristiansen, 1976).

Non-specific binding is a common problem with all immunoadsorbents and polyacrylamide has been recommended instead of Sepharose immunoadsorbents for isolation of detergent solubilized membrane antigens (Haustein and Warr, 1976).

Columns of adsorbents prepared from non-immune immunoglobulins may be used in series with the immunoadsorbent columns to remove non-specific binding species. Subsequently the non-specific components and antigen of interest can be eluted and analysed by polyacrylamide gel electrophoresis in the presence of sodium dodecyl sulphate. Prefiltration through Sepharose alone can be sufficient to remove some contaminants (Fig. 25). Alternatively a preparation containing antigen may be passed through non-immmune IgG-Sepharose columns either before or after elution from the immunoadsorbent in order to remove non-specific binding species. The antigen of interest may be lost to some extent by binding to the non-immune immunoglobulin supports. It is possible that non-specific binding may be considerably reduced by the use of immunoadsorbents prepared with specific antibodies to the antigen of interest. An example of the use of specific antibodies to casein in immunoaffinity chromatography is shown in Fig. 26.

The casein immunoadsorbent was used in conditions where non-specific binding was minimized so that it became the method of choice rather than immunoprecipitation where coprecipitation may complicate interpretation of the data. This is clearly shown with the casein-antibody system in Fig. 26 where analysis of material eluted from immunoadsorbent (Fig. 26a) by polyacrylamide gel electrophoresis in the presence of sodium dodecyl sulphate gives a much clearer picture of the incorporation into the subunits of the antigen than analysis of immunoprecipitates (Fig. 26b). The incorporation into casein after immunoprecipitation and electrophoretic analysis cannot be accurately measured in spite of the fact that the specific anti-casein antibodies (prepared by immunoadsorption, Al-Sarraj *et al.*, 1978) were used for the procedure.

The kinetics for optimal binding of an antigen to an immunoadsorbent

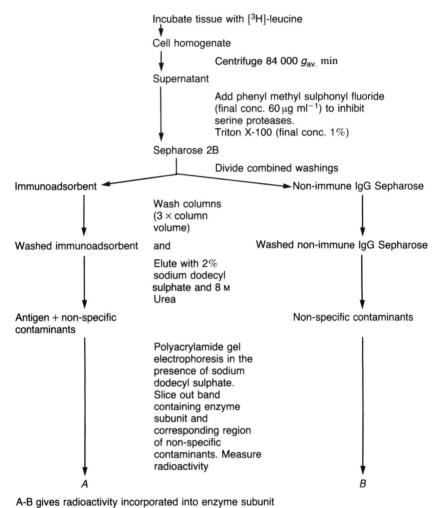

Incubate tissue with [³H]-leucine

Cell homogenate

Centrifuge 84 000 $g_{av.}$ min

Supernatant

Add phenyl methyl sulphonyl fluoride
(final conc. 60 µg ml⁻¹) to inhibit
serine proteases.
Triton X-100 (final conc. 1%)

Sepharose 2B

Divide combined washings

Immunoadsorbent ← → Non-immune IgG Sepharose

Wash columns
(3 × column
volume)

Washed immunoadsorbent   and   Washed non-immune IgG Sepharose

Elute with 2%
sodium dodecyl
sulphate and 8 M
Urea

Antigen + non-specific
contaminants   Non-specific contaminants

Polyacrylamide gel
electrophoresis in the
presence of sodium
dodecyl sulphate.
Slice out band
containing enzyme
subunit and
corresponding region
of non-specific
contaminants. Measure
radioactivity

A   B

A-B gives radioactivity incorporated into enzyme subunit

Fig. 25. Isolation of fatty acid synthetase by immunoadsorbent chromatography.

must be determined with respect to time taken for antigen binding and with respect to the pH and ionic strength of the tissue extract. This is especially important for detergent-solubilized membrane antigens which may show complex binding characteristics to immunoadsorbents.

As a general rule it appears that the binding of soluble antigens (i.e. enzymes or proteins) to immunoadsorbents is more rapid than the binding of detergent solubilized membrane antigens. Further, the binding of

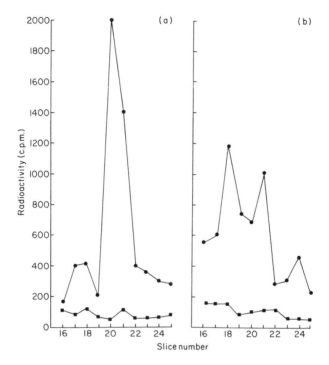

Fig. 26. Polyacrylamide gel electrophoresis of radiolabelled casein isolated by immunoadsorbent chromatography and immunoprecipitation. (a) Samples (0·06–0·4 ml) of particle-free supernatant fractions obtained from mammary explants cultured for 24 h with hormones were applied to either (i) a Sepharose-anti-casein column (3 ml, ●) or (ii) a Sepharose control serum IgG column (3 ml, ■) and left in contact with the column overnight at 4°C. Radiolabelled casein was eluted from the columns with 2%-sodium dodecyl sulphate containing 8 M Urea, dialysed against, water, freeze dried and taken up in sample buffer containing 50 μg of casein (carrier) for electrophoresis. The position of the radioactive peak corresponds to the R_f of purified recombined casein. (b) Samples (0·06–0·4 ml) of particle-free supernatant fractions were mixed with either (i) 1 ml of anti-casein IgG (●) or (ii) 1 ml of control serum IgG (■), and the mixture was incubated for 48 h at 4°C. The immunoprecipitate was washed and processed for electrophoresis as described above.

detergent-solubilized membrane antigens can be considerably influenced by detergent type and concentration. This might be expected in view of the micellar composition of detergent solutions and equilibria which may exist between different micellar forms of an antigen which may expose more or less antigenic determinants.

The binding of purified fatty acid synthetase to an immunoadsorbent is complete in 5–10 min at room temperature (Fig. 27). Acetyl-CoA carboxylase binds to its immunoadsorbent in a similarly short time. The binding of enzymes in detergent solubilized extracts of mitochondrial preparations

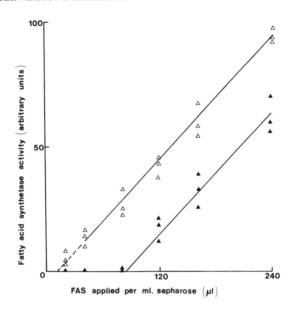

Fig. 27. Binding of fatty acid synthetase (FAS) activity to columns of non-immune IgG-Sepharose or (anti-FAS)-IgG-Sepharose. Purified FAS in 0·25 M phosphate buffer, pH 7·0 was applied to 1·0 ml columns of either non-immune IgG-Sepharose or (anti-FAS)-IgG-Sepharose. After 5–10 min, the columns were eluted with 3 ml of the same buffer and aliquots of the eluate were assayed for FAS activity. Activity binding to non-immune IgG-Sepharose columns (△); activity binding to (anti-FAS)-IgG-Sepharose columns (▲). The results with three series of columns are shown.

show very different binding characteristics to their respective immunoadsorbents (Fig. 28). The binding of cytochrome oxidase is completed over a period of two hours, that of monoamine oxidase is only completed after overnight incubation, while pyruvate dehydrogenase binding is complete after 15–30 min. Pyruvate dehydrogenase is called a "soluble" mitochondrial enzyme although it is very difficult to remove from mitochondrial preparations without detergent. The behaviour of this enzyme in detergent (cholate) is very similar to other soluble enzymes, i.e. rapid binding to immunoadsorbent (Fig. 28c).

Cytochrome oxidase binding from a cholate solution (Fig. 28a) is similar to that seen when the enzyme is dissolved in Triton X-100 (Walker and Mayer, 1977). If the enzyme is left in contact with the immunoadsorbent for 2·5 h at room temperature the binding characteristics are identical to those shown by soluble enzymes in much shorter periods of time, e.g. 10–15 min (cf. Fig. 29 and Fig. 27). Monoamine oxidase shows much slower binding to its immunoadsorbent than does cytochrome oxidase (Fig. 28b) although both enzymes were solubilized by the same detergent under

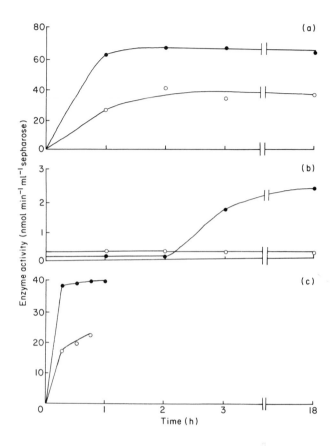

Fig. 28. Binding characteristics of immunoadsorbents with antigens in detergent solution. Mitochondrial preparations were solubilized in 20 mM sodium phosphate buffer, pH 7·4 containing 1% (w/v) sodium cholate. The detergent solubilized material was preincubated with Sepharose 4B for 30 min at room temperature before application to the immunoadsorbents. The Sepharose 4B was washed with three volumes of the buffer and the combined washings were used for enzyme immunoisolation. Samples of the combined washings were applied to Sepharose 4B immunoadsorbents (prepared by the cyanogen bromide method) containing antibodies to cytochrome oxidase (a), monoamine oxidase (b) and pyruvate dehydrogenase (c) and incubated at room temperature. The binding of the immunoadsorbent for cytochrome oxidase was measured with antibody excess whereas binding to the other immunoadsorbents was estimated with antigen excess. Immunoglobulin G containing antibodies of interest was used to prepare immunoadsorbents to cytochrome oxidase and pyruvate dehydrogenase whereas purified antibodies (prepared by mitochondrial adsorption; Fig. 6) were used to prepare the immunoadsorbent to monoamine oxidase. Both immunoadsorbent (●) and non-immune IgG-Sepharose (○) used for the isolation of cytochrome oxidase, monoamine oxidase, and pyruvate dehydrogenase contained 10 mg, 0·2 mg and 10 mg of bound protein per millilitre of Sepharose respectively.

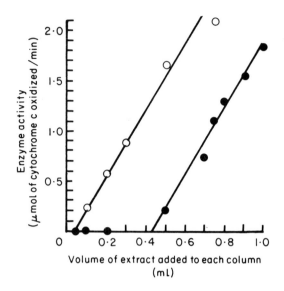

Fig 29. Binding of cytochrome oxidase to an immunoadsorbent after prolonged contact. Samples of a mitochondrial Triton X-100 (1%, v/v) extract were left in contact with the columns for 2·5 h at room tenmperature. Enzyme activity washed off non-immune IgG-Sepharose column (○), enzyme activity washed off antiserum-Sepharose column (●).

identical conditions. The only difference was that purified antibodies to monoamine oxidase were used for the preparation of its immunoadsorbent (Fig. 6).

Non-specific binding of the enzymes to non-immune IgG-Sepharose is apparently a function of the concentration of coupled protein since both the non-immune IgG-Sepharose preparations used for cytochrome oxidase and pyruvate dehydrogenase had 10 mg protein per millilitre and bound considerable enzyme activity non-specifically, whereas the non-immune IgG-Sepharose used with monoamine oxidase has 0·2 mg protein per millilitre and bound no enzyme activity.

Many elution systems have been described for immunoadsorbents (Ruoslahti, 1976) where extremes of pH or ionic strength have been often used. These conditions alone are not always sufficient to elute an antigen of interest. Complete elution of acetyl-CoA carboxylase, fatty acid synthetase and cytochrome oxidase from their respective immunoadsorbents can only be achieved with 8 M urea containing 2% (w/v) sodium dodecyl sulphate (Table 3; Walker, Paskin, Manning and Mayer, unpublished observations). Fortunately, when measuring incorporation of radioactive amino acids into protein antigens it is not necessary to preserve the conformation of the antigen on elution from the immunoadsorbent.

Table 3
Elution of antigens from immunoadsorbents

Immunoadsorbent for	Acetyl-CoA carboxylase	Fatty acid synthetase	Cytochrome oxidase
			Antigen eluted (%)
Eluant			
2·5 M MgCl$_2$	—	—	—
0·2 M Glycine-HCl, pH 2·8	—	7·8	—
8 M Urea	approx. 100	27	20
8 M Urea +2% (w/v) sodium dodecyl sulphate	—	75·3	74

Immunoadsorbents were successively eluted with the eluants.

Elution of immunoadsorbents with urea-sodium dodecyl sulphate brings about a varying degree of loss of binding capacity of the immunoadsorbent. Immunoadsorbents to casein and fatty acid synthetase lose 5–10% of their binding capacity after a single elution with the denaturing solvents. However, an immunoadsorbent to monoamine oxidase loses approximately 50% of binding capacity and an immunoadsorbent to cytochrome oxidase loses approximately 30% of binding capacity during each elution. The best solvents are obviously those which lead to the minimum loss of binding capacity, but which quantitatively elute an antigen.

The use of electrophoretic elution of antigens from immunoadsorbents (Dean et al., 1977) seems to have great potential as a gentle but effective elution technique which does not require denaturing solvents. A convenient apparatus which can be used for this procedure is supplied by ISCO (ISCO Model 1750: sample concentrator. ISCO, Nebraska, USA). This apparatus can be used not only to elute an antigen but to concentrate it at the same time.

Immunoadsorbents can be conveniently used to isolate antigens from biological fluids or tissue extracts. The conditions for immunoadsorption and elution must be carefully established and the recovery of bound antigen must be carefully checked. If these conditions are known then rapid quantitative isolation of an antigen from a tissue extract can be carried out.

If an antigen is to be isolated from a tissue extract without much denaturation then the immunoadsorbent should be prepared with an antiserum containing antibodies with low affinities to the antigen. Under these conditions it might be expected that some compromise may be

Table 4
Immunoprecipitation and immunoadsorption
chromatography: a comparison

Point	Immunoprecipitation	Immunoadsorption chromatography
1a. Non-specific contamination	Co-precipitation	Non-specific adsorption
b. Elimination of non-specifically bound protein	Washing procedures and use of specific antibodies to antigen	Washing and use of specific antibodies to antigen
c. Which method has most contamination?	—	—
2. Carrier enzyme	Usually needed	Not needed usually
3. Protein in immuno-isolated material	Often mostly immunoglobulin	Mostly antigen of interest
4a. Polyacrylamide gel electrophoresis in sodium dodecyl sulphate	Must be carried out	Must be carried out
b. Material applied to gel	Mostly immuno-gloublin	Mostly antigen
5. Simple or complex antigen subunit composition on polyacrylamide gels	Causes problems of interpretation if low radiolabel incorporation (see 4b)	Causes less problems of interpretation of radiolabel incorporation
6. Quantity of antibodies needed	Large quantities can be needed. Depends on amount of carrier used	Low binding capacity and loss of binding capacity can lead to large antibody requirement
7. Rapidity of immunoisolation	Can be made rapid by ultracentri-fugation of immunocomplexes	Extremely rapid with non-membrane antigens; complex slow binding characteristics with detergent solubilized membrane antigens

reached whereby an antigen would bind to an immunoadsorbent and be eluted from the immunoadsorbent in relatively mild conditions.

Finally it should be noted that immunoadsorbents can be very sensitive to antigen modification. Modification of fatty acid synthetase or cytochrome oxidase by mild acetylation or iodination results in the production of species with complex binding and elution properties (Walker, Paskin and Mayer, unpublished observations).

The basic problem for the would-be immunochemist is whether to use immunoprecipitation or immunoaffinity chromatography for isolation of the antigen of interest. There is no short answer to this problem since both methods have advantages and difficulties. The final decision must be influenced by consideration of co-precipitation versus non-specific binding to an immunoadsorbent, the purpose for which the antigen is isolated and the molecular properties of the protein antigen. Some points for consideration are shown in Table 4. As a rather sweeping generalization the immunoaffinity methods are usually of most use to biological scientists intent on rapidly isolating an antigen; however, immunoprecipitation has made, and continues to make, a major contribution in antigen isolation in several fields of biochemistry and molecular biology.

IV. Immunohistochemistry

The "art" of immunohistochemistry has been elegantly described elsewhere (e.g. Poole, 1974; Sternberger, 1974). These intricate and beautiful techniques are generally outside the scope of this book, although biological scientists should be encouraged to find out whether these methods are applicable to their immunochemical problem. Antisera of very low titre are routinely used to give good results with immunohistochemical techniques. For example, an antiserum to chromomembrin B (Winkler et al., 1974) which could only be shown to interact with the antigen by means of microcomplement fixation, gave good results when used as the peroxidase-conjugate to locate the membrane antigen. Similarly in clinical immunochemistry, human sera are routinely assayed for auto-antibodies by immunofluorescent localization of antigens in tissue preparations from experimental animals. For immunofluorescence studies antibodies may be labelled in several ways including conjugation with fluorescein or rhodamine.

Peroxidase conjugated antibodies are also frequently used. Here the conjugate is visualized by allowing the peroxidase moiety to oxidize diaminobenzidine in the presence of hydrogen peroxide. The resulting oxidation product reacts strongly with osmium tetroxide to produce a brown/black stain which may be observed with a light or electron microscope.

In many fields of biology ferritin-conjugated antibodies are used in conjugation with the electron microscope to study membrane antigens.

These elegant techniques deserve special mention since they have been used to give exciting information on the structure of intracellular membranes.

A. Ferritin-conjugated Antibodies

Increasingly cell biologists are wanting to know the vectorial orientation of proteins in cell membranes. Interest ranges widely from studies on the general protein topography of some specific membrane to studies on the functional characteristics and molecular properties of proteins on one side of a membrane or another. It is quite apparent that until we know these topological features of membrane proteins we will not understand, for example, membrane synthesis and degradation or the functional interactions of cells with their environment by means of membrane receptors for hormones, neurotransmitters and other exogenous molecules.

In the next section the value of immunoinhibition titrations in determining the vectorial orientation of enzymes is described and some of the theoretical and practical problems are outlined. Unfortunately immunoinhibition of membrane enzymes is often incomplete or has complex characteristics and therefore an alternative technique must be sought in order to corroborate or improve on the results from these methods.

Several investigators have chosen to study topographical localization of proteins by means of the use of ferritin-conjugated antibodies and electron microscopy, the iron-loaded ferritin conjugate acting as an electron-dense probe for some membrane antigen. The approach may be divided into three parts: the preparation of the ferritin-antibody conjugate, the mixing of the conjugate with the membrane preparation and the preparation of the samples for electron microscopy.

Choice of conjugate has varied in different laboratories. Some workers have used ferritin conjugated with immunoaffinity purified specific antibodies (perhaps the ideal method) whereas others have used ferritin conjugated to IgG containing antibodies to the antigen of interest. A novel choice of conjugate has been "hybrid" antibodies consisting of antibodies to the antigen of interest and ferritin which in turn is coupled to ferritin. The whole complex is then used as the membrane probe.

Ferritin-antibody complexes can be used in two different methods: either ferritin conjugated to the antibody of interest (the direct method) or ferritin conjugated to antibodies prepared to immunoglobulin from the animal species in which antibodies to the antigen of interest were raised (the indirect method). It has been argued that the direct method is better since it gives in certain cases better resolution and quantitatively better results (Matsura *et al.*, 1978).

It is obviously impossible to describe all the variations in technique which have been described in the literature but details of the methods described above will be presented in Figs 30–32. The use of ferritin-conjugated antibodies is undoubtedly an excellent approach to the study of membrane topography of proteins.

1. Ferritin-conjugated antibodies: the direct method of use. An example is given of the use of ferritin-conjugated antibodies in the localization of cytochrome c oxidase in the mitochondrial inner membrane (Hackenbrock and Hammon, 1975). Antibodies to cytochrome oxidase were purified

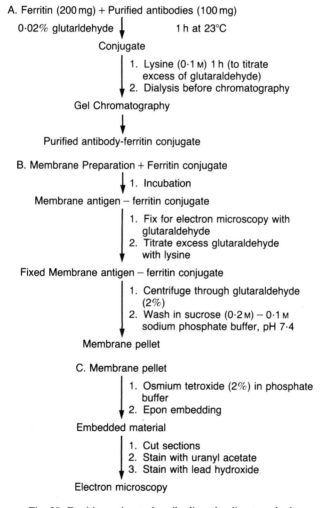

Fig. 30. Ferritin-conjugated antibodies: the direct method.

from IgG by immunoadsorption chromatography with Sepharose-cytochrome c oxidase. The ferritin was coupled to the specific antibodies with glutaraldehyde and the ferritin-antibody conjugate was separated by gel filtration from unconjugated ferritin, unconjugated antibodies and polymerized material. The scheme for preparation and use of the conjugate is shown in Fig. 30. Titration of excess glutaraldehyde can be achieved with amino acids, e.g. lysine (Fig. 30) or glycine (Matsura *et al.*, 1978) and the antibody-ferritin ratio of the final preparation can be measured, e.g. after immunoaffinity chromatography on Sepharose-antigen (Matsura *et al.*, 1978). The conditions for use of the conjugate depend on the nature of the organelle or membrane preparation, e.g. its susceptibility to lysis and can therefore vary from a few minutes (Hackenbrock and Hammon, 1975) to prolonged periods (Matsura *et al.*, 1978).

The successful use of ferritin-antibody conjugate depends on the choice of good controls to assess non-specific binding of the conjugate and therefore spurious electron dense areas on the membrane surface. Non-specific binding of antibody and ferritin in the conjugate to the membrane surface must be checked. This can be done by preincubating membrane preparations with antibody or ferritin followed by the conjugate (Hackenbrock and Hammon, 1975) or by incubating membrane fractions with a conjugate prepared from non-immune IgG and ferritin (Matsura *et al.*, 1978). When IgG ferritin conjugate, rather than specific antibody conjugate is used, a further control showing that binding is due to antibody conjugate and not adventitious protein ferritin conjugate may be carried out: the antigen is mixed with the conjugate and the extent of binding of any ferritin to membranes from this mixture estimated.

2. Ferritin-conjugated antibodies: the indirect method of use. In this approach the conjugate is prepared with ferritin and antibodies to immunoglobulin from the animal species in which antibodies to the antigen of interest were raised. Antibodies for ferritin coupling may be raised to IgG or to F_{ab} fragments prepared from the IgG (Morimoto *et al.*, 1976). The preparation and use of the conjugate is shown in Fig. 31 (Morimoto *et al.*, 1976). These authors report that the conjugate retains 30–50% of antibody titre and behaves like monovalent antibodies.

There are two immunochemical reactions, both of which must be controlled. The first reaction can be controlled by the addition of non-immune IgG instead of IgG containing antibodies to the antigen of interest. The second reaction can be prevented by replacing the ferritin-antibody conjugate with ferritin non-immune IgG. Alternatively the interaction of the ferritin conjugate with the membrane-antibody complex can be prevented by addition of non-conjugated second antibody. All these controls minimize misinterpretation of electron microscopic data.

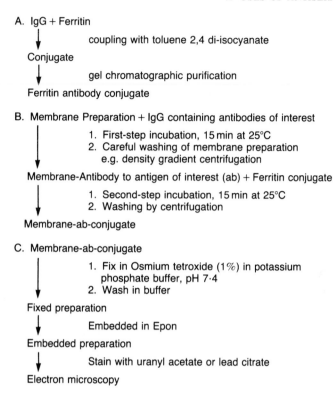

A. IgG + Ferritin

↓   coupling with toluene 2,4 di-isocyanate

Conjugate

↓   gel chromatographic purification

Ferritin antibody conjugate

B. Membrane Preparation + IgG containing antibodies of interest

↓
     1. First-step incubation, 15 min at 25°C
     2. Careful washing of membrane preparation
        e.g. density gradient centrifugation

Membrane-Antibody to antigen of interest (ab) + Ferritin conjugate

↓
     1. Second-step incubation, 15 min at 25°C
     2. Washing by centrifugation

Membrane-ab-conjugate

C. Membrane-ab-conjugate

↓
     1. Fix in Osmium tetroxide (1%) in potassium
        phosphate buffer, pH 7·4
     2. Wash in buffer

Fixed preparation

↓   Embedded in Epon

Embedded preparation

↓   Stain with uranyl acetate or lead citrate

Electron microscopy

Fig. 31. Ferritin-conjugated antibodies: the indirect method.

3. *"Hybrid" antibody-ferritin conjugates.* A section of ferritin-conjugated antibodies would be incomplete without reference to a method which deserves mention for novelty as well as its use in the elucidation of the vectorial orientation of cytochrome b_5 (Remacle *et al.*, 1974). The method consists of the preparation of hybrid antibodies (i.e. to antigen and ferritin by means of the method of Nisonoff and Palmer, 1964). The hybrid antibodies were purified by immunoaffinity chromatography and coupled to ferritin by simple mixing. After removal of excess ferritin the conjugate was ready for use (Fig. 32). Controls were carried out by mixing a large excess of antigen with the conjugate before use with the membrane fraction.

V. Recent Developments in the Uses of Antibodies

Increasingly greater imagination is being put into the use of immunoche-mical techniques, either through new serological developments or by the

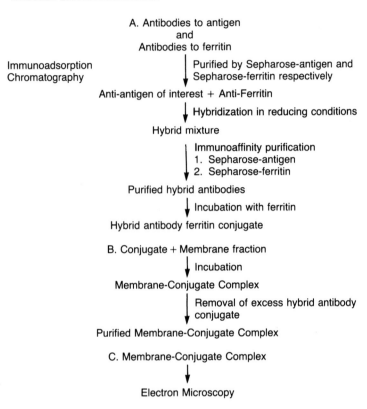

A. Antibodies to antigen
and
Antibodies to ferritin

Immunoadsorption
Chromatography

Purified by Sepharose-antigen and
Sepharose-ferritin respectively

Anti-antigen of interest + Anti-Ferritin

Hybridization in reducing conditions

Hybrid mixture

Immunoaffinity purification
1. Sepharose-antigen
2. Sepharose-ferritin

Purified hybrid antibodies

Incubation with ferritin

Hybrid antibody ferritin conjugate

B. Conjugate + Membrane fraction

Incubation

Membrane-Conjugate Complex

Removal of excess hybrid antibody
conjugate

Purified Membrane-Conjugate Complex

C. Membrane-Conjugate Complex

Electron Microscopy

Fig. 32. Hybrid antibody-ferritin conjugates.

use of existing immunochemical techniques in conjugation with developments in other fields of biological science. Therefore under the heading of recent developments in the uses of antibodies will be described a variety of new procedures for the study of soluble and membrane protein antigens. These techniques serve to illustrate the increasing usefulness of immunochemical procedures in different fields of biological science.

A. Antibodies as Membrane Surface Probes

It becomes increasingly apparent that the vectorial orientation of enzymes and proteins in cellular membranes is not random but strictly ordered. Proteins may be found on the cytoplasmic or internal surface of intracellular organelles and on the cytoplasmic or external surface of the plasma membrane. Much work has been carried out on the orientation of proteins in the plasma membrane: it has been shown that proteins do not cross from one side of the cell membrane to the other but that lateral flow of proteins on the inside or outside of the cell membrane commonly occurs (Rothman and Lenard, 1977). Many proteins and protein complexes (e.g. cytochrome oxidase) are transmembraneous; this is presumably related to their functions in transporting molecules or generating potential gradients across membranes. Orientation is again absolute, with distinctive domains or subunits being found on one side of the membrane or the other. Recently the curious distribution of an enzyme, apparently on both sides of the mitochondrial outer membrane, has been presented (Russell *et al.*, 1978a). Similarly, subunits of an enzyme complex (i.e. cytochrome oxidase) may be on both sides of the mitochondrial inner membrane (Chan and Tracy, 1978). This raises several problems, some relating to the doctrines described above, others particularly concerning the molecular nature of the enzyme at each site (e.g. covalent modifications) and the biosynthetic problems involved in the biomodal distribution of the enzyme.

Most of the information on the vectorial orientation of proteins in membranes comes from the use of chemical reagents which are defined as reacting with proteins on one surface of a membrane only and therefore specifying the position of proteins on the membrane (Marchesi and Furthmayr, 1976). The main problem with chemical reagents relates to the possibility that they will cross the membrane and therefore invalidate interpretation of the results. Attempts have been made to minimize this problem with the use of reactive intermediates generated by large enzymes which are presumed not to cross membranes (e.g. lactoperoxidase catalysed iodination of cell surface or organelle membrane proteins). Even this development lacks the ultimate preference which is molecular specificity of the modifying reagent. Modified membrane proteins must be analysed in some way in order to characterize the orientation of some known enzyme or protein. This must involve some method of purification of the protein of interest. Chemical surface probes have often provided useful information in a general sense, e.g. on the fraction of proteins in a cell membrane which are exposed externally or which are glycosylated. However, the vectorial orientation of specific proteins must be known to understand their functional or turnover characteristics.

Antibodies to an enzyme or protein should theoretically, answer many of these problems since specificity should be absolute and antibody molecules are so large that they will not transverse membranes (except by endocytosis). Indeed, antisera to membrane components have been used for many years to characterize cell surfaces: immunohistochemical techniques have proved excellent for characterizing cell types or specific components in cell surfaces (see previous section).

1. Immunoinhibition to determine enzyme orientation. Antibodies can be used to identify the vectorial orientation of enzymes in membranes by means of their immunoinhibitory capacity. The immunoinhibition of enzyme activity can be used as evidence that an enzyme is accessible to the antibodies: this can be used to define the orientation of an enzyme in a cell membrane or organelle surface. The reasons for immunoinhibition of a membrane enzyme must be complex: the phenomenon is not simply the result of the presence of anti-catalytic antibodies (often present in small quantities in antisera due to evolutionary conservation of catalytic sites, Cinader, 1977), but must also depend on conformational distortions, which are a function of the number of accessible immunodeterminants on the exposed surface of the enzyme.

Problems which may be encountered in the use of immunochemical probes of membrane orientation of enzymes are illustrated by studies on monoamine oxidase (Russell *et al.*, 1978a). This enzyme is found in the outer mitochondrial membrane but its orientation is unknown. The basic principle in the use of antibodies to the enzyme (prepared by partial adsorption, Fig. 6) is that the distribution of the enzyme can be calculated from the fraction of the enzyme immunoinhibited in iso-osmotic and hypo-osmotic conditions. In the latter conditions the mitochondrial outer membrane will rupture, thus allowing access of antibodies to any enzyme which may be present on the inside of the outer membrane. Naturally if an enzyme is present on only one side of a membrane all or none of its activity may be inhibited depending on whether it is on the outside or inside respectively. Trans-membraneous enzymes should be inhibited theoretically by antibodies presented at either membrane surface. This technique can be performed for enzymes or proteins on any cell membrane which can be subjected to osmotic lysis (e.g. plasma membrane, mitochondrial inner and outer membranes, microsomal membranes).

There are several assumptions and difficulties with the experimental design which are obviously applicable to studies on other membrane enzymes besides monoamine oxidase. The basic assumptions are that all the enzyme activity is assayed in all mitochondrial preparations and that the sum of enzyme activity on the outside (E_O) and inside (E_I) of the membrane accounts for all the enzyme activity, i.e.

$$E_O + E_I = 1$$

After incubation with control serum under identical conditions to anti-serum the enzyme activity remaining (C_S) is given by:

$$E_O + E_I = C_S$$

There are two major difficulties with the application of this method to monoamine oxidase. First the enzyme has multiple substrate specificities and the different activities (i.e. towards β-phenyl ethylamine, tyramine and 5-hydroxytryptamine) are inhibited incompletely and to different extents by the antiserum. These observations are made on detergent solubilized enzyme (Fig. 33) and on membrane-bound enzyme: the maximum immunoinhibition of the membrane-bound enzyme in mitochondrial preparations was different from the solubilized enzyme, being 40% for β-phenylethylamine, 37% for tyramine and 27% for 5-hydroxytryptamine.

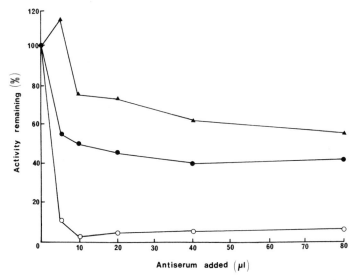

Fig. 33. Immunotitration of monoamine oxidase activities in detergent extracts of mitochondrial preparations from human liver. Samples (20 μl) of Triton X-100-depleted (with Biobeads SM-2) Triton X-100 extracts of human liver mitochondrial preparations were incubated overnight at 4°C with antiserum. Protein concentrations were kept constant in all samples by the addition of bovine serum albumin. The activities are expressed after correction for non-specific inhibition as measured with control serum. Enzyme activities were assayed with β-phenylethylamine (▲), tyramine (●) and 5-hydroxytrypamine (○).

The reason for this difference is not clear but presumably results from the different exposure of antigenic determinants in the solubilized and membrane-bound enzyme (Hackenbrock and Hammon, 1975). In order to carry out a calculation of the vectorial distribution of the enzyme activities it must be assumed that a constant proportion of the accessible enzyme is immunoinhibited in unlysed and lysed mitochondrial preparations (i.e. in iso-osmotic and hypo-osmotic conditions). This assumption is verified since a constant proportion of each enzyme activity (i.e. the proportion described above) was immunoinhibited in all mitochondrial preparations. Obviously a factor for incomplete inhibition must be included in a calculation of enzyme distribution.

The second difficulty is that preparations of so-called unlysed mitochondria in iso-osmotic conditions in fact contain lysed mitochondria. Therefore, a measure of the degree of mitochondrial lysis in both iso- and hypo-osmotic conditions must be obtained. This is conveniently carried out by measuring the fraction of an intermembrane space marker (adenylate kinase) which is susceptible to trypsin digestion in iso- and hypo-osmotic conditions.

Before describing the calculation it is worth noting that these complications were unexpected and illustrate the problems which might occur in the use of antibodies as membrane probes. However, these empirical observations have suggested principles which can be used for studies on all membrane enzymes.

The calculation of the vectorial orientation of the forms of monoamine oxidase which catalyse the oxidation of β-phenylethylamine, tyramine and 5-hydroxytryptamine in human liver mitochondrial preparations are as follows:

2. In iso-osmotic conditions. The fraction of each enzyme activity remaining after immunoinhibition, i.e. E_{AS}/E_{CS} should be E_I where E_{AS} = monoamine oxidase activity (defined by each substrate) after incubation with antiserum and E_{CS} = monoamine oxidase activity (defined by each substrate) remaining after incubation with control serum. However, (i) all activity is not immunoinhibited and (ii) iso-osmotic mitochondrial preparations are lysed to some extent.

Therefore the fraction of enzyme activity remaining after incubation with excess antiserum

$$= E_R{}^{IS} = XE_O + (1-F_1)E_I + XF_1E_I \tag{1}$$

where X = fraction of enzyme activity which is not immunoinhibited and F_1 = fraction of lysed mitochondria.

3. In hypo-osmotic conditions. Fraction of enzyme activity remaining after incubation with excess antiserum

$$= E_R{}^H = XE_O + (1-F_2)E_I + XF_2E_I \tag{2}$$

where F_2 = fraction of lysed mitochondria.

Therefore
$$E_R{}^{IS} - E_R{}^H = E_I(F_2-F_1) - X(F_2-F_1) \tag{3}$$
$$= E_I(1-X)(F_2-F_1) \tag{4}$$

Therefore
$$E_I = \frac{E_R{}^{IS} - E_R{}^H}{(1-X)(F_2-F_1)} \tag{5}$$

and $E_O = 1 - E_I.$ \hfill (6)

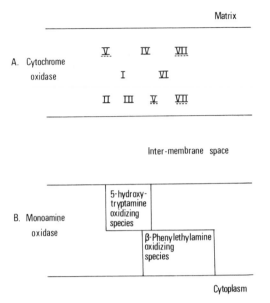

Fig. 34. Vectorial orientation of mitochondrial enzymes shown by immunochemical analysis.
A. Orientation of cytochrome oxidase subunits as studied with antisera to subunits V and VII.
B. Orientation of monoamine oxidase as studied with a mitochondrially adsorbed antiserum to the enzyme (see Fig. 6).

By means of these calculations (i.e. equations (5) and (6)) it can be shown for human liver mitochondrial preparations that immunochemically accessible monoamine oxidase is present on both sides of the outer mitochondrial membrane, and that the form of the enzyme oxidizing β-phenylethylamine is present on the outer surface, while the form of the enzyme oxidizing 5-hydroxytryptamine is present on the inner surface of the membrane.

In spite of the difficulties the use of antisera as membrane-impermeable probes of the structure and function of membranes, by methods other than those involving immunohistochemical techniques is to be recommended. Such approaches will help to define membrane topography without the problems associated with the use of chemical reagents, although a multi-technique attack on the problem will probably give the most meaningful results. This is illustrated by the many approaches used to study the orientation of cytochrome oxidase in the mitochondrial inner membrane (e.g. Chan and Tracy, 1978). The proposed orientation of cytochrome oxidase and monoamine oxidase in the inner and outer mitochondrial membranes respectively as demonstrated by immunochemical techniques are shown in Fig. 34.

4. Immunoadsorption to study vectorial orientation of antigens. (a) The method of Jørgensen (1976) utilized an anti-synaptosomal antiserum produced in rabbits. The principle of the method was to incubate synaptosomes or lysed synaptosomes with the antiserum. After incubation both types of synaptosomes were solubilized in 2% (v/v) Triton X–100 and subjected to a first dimension line immunoelectrophoresis (Krøll, 1973b),

1. Preliminary incubation (e.g. in iso-osmotic conditions)

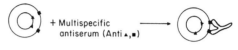

2. Degergent solubilization

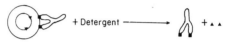

3. Crossed immunoelectrophoresis

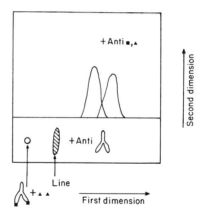

Fig. 35. Immunoadsorption to study vectorial orientation.

and then a second dimension immunoelectrophoresis. The first dimension contained pig antibodies to rabbit immunoglobulins while the second dimension contained rabbit anti-synaptosomal antibodies. Any antigens which reacted with anti-synaptosomal antibodies in the preliminary incubation would be precipitated as a line in the first dimension electrophoresis while antigens which did not react should be precipitated in the second dimension electrophoresis. Identification of the orientation of antigens was made easier by carrying out the preliminary incubations in iso-osmotic or hypo-osmotic conditions at several antibody concentrations. Progressive diappearance of an antigen immunoprecipitate from the second dimension of the immunoelectrophoresis could, therefore, be used to clearly identify the orientation of the specific antigen. The principle of the method is shown in Fig. 35.

(b)   The method of Bjerrum *et al.* (1975) involves adsorbing samples of a polyspecific antiserum with intact or lysed cell or organelle membrane preparations. The adsorbed antisera can then be tested against detergent extracts of the cell or organelle membrane preparation in order to identify antigens which face inside or outside or which may be transmembranous in the cell or organelle preparation. The disadvantage of the method, compared to that of Jørgensen, is that far greater amounts of cells or organelles are required for the procedure.

Both of these methods can be performed with monospecific antisera in order to locate specific antigens of interest.

B. Determination of Antigen Molecular Weight

The molecular weight of an uncharacterized antigen may be determined by immunochemical analysis following separation of the antigen on calibrated gel filtration columns (Svendsen, 1973). The immunoisolated antigen can be analysed by polyacrylamide gel electrophoresis in the presence of sodium dodecyl sulphate in order to determine the molecular weight of the antigen subunit(s) (Ross *et al.*, 1978). As previously mentioned (Chapter 3) highly radioactive antigen mixtures (labelled *in vivo* or *in vitro*) may be analysed with polyspecific antisera by cross-rocket immunoelectrophoresis. The individual rockets can be analysed by polyacrylamide gel electrophoresis in the presence of sodium dodecyl sulphate (Norrild *et al.*, 1977; Walker, unpublished observations; Fig. 4). The individual subunits may be visualized by autoradiography, fluorography or, alternatively, radioactivity may be estimated by gel slicing and scintillation counting.

C. Determination of Antigen Isoelectric Point

For many antigens it may be possible to determine isoelectric point by means of crossed-rocket immunoelectrophoresis with isoelectric focusing in the first dimension (Söderholm *et al.*, 1975). This method may also work for antigens separated in the presence of urea. For antigens labelled *in vivo* individual immunoprecipitates from crossed-rocket immunoelectrophoresis may be analysed by isoelectric focusing in the presence of 8 M urea in a manner analogous to that described above for the determination of antigen subunit molecular weight.

If a monospecific antiserum is available it is possible to analyse non-radioactive immunoprecipitates directly by means of two-dimensional electrophoresis and thus determine the isoelectric point and molecular weight of the antigen at the same time. This method has been used to distinguish the presence of modified forms of hypoxanthine phosphoribosyltransferase in Lesch–Nyhan syndrome (Ghangas and Milman, 1977).

D. Determination of the Intrinsic or Extrinsic Nature of Membrane Proteins

Charge-shift electrophoresis of membrane proteins (Helenius and Simons, 1977) distinguishes intrinsic membrane proteins from extrinsic membrane proteins or cytosolic proteins on the basis of the interaction of these proteins with charged and non-ionic detergents. Only the intrinsic membrane proteins bind both types of detergent and thus only they show an alteration in their electrophoretic mobilities. By using charge-shift electrophoresis as a first dimension separation technique in crossed-immunoelectrophoresis it is possible to characterize membrane protein antigens in terms of their amphiphilic nature (Jørgensen, 1977).

E. Identification of Calcium-binding Proteins

The mobility of Ca^{2+}-binding proteins on agarose gel electrophoresis depends greatly upon whether calcium is bound to the protein. Binding of Ca^{2+} greatly reduces the mobility of the protein and thus immunoelectrophoretic analysis with first dimension electrophoresis in the presence of Ca^{2+} or EDTA may be used to demonstrate if a protein binds Ca^{2+} (Suttie et al., 1977).

F. Identification of Phosphorylated Antigens

Gordon et al. (1977a,b) and Teichberg et al. (1977) have combined crossed immunoelectrophoresis with in vitro phosphorylation of membrane proteins to demonstrate that the 65 000 dalton subunit of acetylcholine receptor is phosphorylated when membranes are incubated for short periods with ^{32}P-ATP.

Similarly crossed immunoelectrophoresis of casein samples gives a complex pattern of connected rockets, probably due to different degrees of phosphorylation of the different forms of the protein (Fig. 8).

G. *Isolation of Specific Cell Types and Subcellular Organelles*

The subfractionation of B and T lymphocytes by means of anti IgG serum is sufficiently well characterized to have found its way into textbooks of practical immunology (e.g. Hudson and Hay, 1976). Similar subfraction schemes should be possible, in principle, for all cell types which possess characteristic antigenic determinants. Similarly the subfractionation of subcellular organelles by means of antisera to specific surface antigens on each organelle should also be feasilble. This is especially important in cases where heterogeneous populations of the same type of organelle are present (e.g. synaptic vesicles containing different transmitters, see Chapter 6) or where a particular type of subcellular organelle is present in a variety of forms (e.g. the plasma membrane which on homogenization gives rise to sheets and vesicles). An immunological procedure for the isolation of plasma membranes has been developed (Luzio *et al.*, 1976) and by the use of a double antibody technique, enabled specific purification of those membrane vesicles with "outside-out" conformation. Without the use of a double-antibody technique the authors could not obtain a purification equivalent to that obtained by conventional subcellular fractionation techniques.

5

Case Study I: Immunological Studies on Membrane Protein Antigens

In previous sections the value of immunochemical reagents as probes of the membrane surface have been discussed, specifically with reference to the use of immunoinhibition and immunoadsorption to determine membrane topography and the use of immunoreagents in electron microscopy (Chapter 4). These specific uses of antisera to membrane proteins are but a few examples of the use of immunochemical probes which are described in the literature.

The purpose of this case study is to illustrate the widely differing potential of immunochemical reagents for the study of cell membranes. The precise structural and functional attributes of all cellular membranes must be known before cellular dynamics can be understood. Immunochemical techniques can be used to study most of the problems related to membrane proteins. Studies of a great number of problems relating to membrane proteins are shown in Table 5.

As mentioned elsewhere, it is not the intention to be completely comprehensive in analysis of the literature but simply to use some reported information to illustrate the usefulness and diversity of immunochemical techniques. The specific intentions of this study on membrane antigens are to illustrate the diverse uses of immunochemical reagents; to show areas where much effort has been exerted, and hopefully, to give indications of where immunochemical techniques may be profitably used in the future.

The nature of each problem shown in Table 5 will be described in more detail to show precisely the reasons for the use of the immunochemical approach. The technical and methodological enterprise used to tackle the different problems will be described in tabular form (Table 6) so that the reader can note the innovation which many workers have used in order to

Table 5
Membrane problems subjected to immunochemical analysis

1. Vectorial orientation of membrane proteins
2. Characterization of specific membrane enzymology
3. Sites of synthesis of membrane proteins
4. Turnover of membrane proteins
5. Resolution of metabolic pathways
6. Functional interactions of membrane enzymes
7. Functional and morphological heterogeneity in defined cell membranes
8. Functional and morphological homology of proteins in different tissues and species
9. Functional and structural interrelationships of parts of protein complexes
10. Conformational pertubation of membrane proteins
11. Degree of exposure of membrane proteins
12. Proximity of membrane proteins
13. Orientation of membrane vesicles
14. Changes in membrane enzymology in carcinogenesis
15. Changes in membrane proteins in tumours

exploit the immunochemical approach successfully. This method of presentation of data (Table 6) is grouped under subheadings defined by subcellular organization rather than biological problem. In this way the reader can see how each biomembrane system may pose novel or general problems for immunochemical solution.

I. Membrane Problems Subjected to Immunochemical Analysis

The problems in Table 5 are those which have been subjected to immunochemical analysis. In general the problems outlined include most areas of current research on membrane proteins. It is clear that immunochemical reagents have played a key role in elucidation of some of these problems. The techniques which have been developed offer new probes of membrane structure and function which can be used in all fields of biomedical science.

The topography of cell membranes, specifically with respect to the vectorial orientation of membrane proteins and the consequent asymmetry of membrane functions has been studied extensively by immunochemical techniques. Here antibodies are used as membrane-impermeable reagents, which can be used to decide whether a protein is transmembranous or whether it resides on one side of a membrane or the other. A variety of analytical techniques (e.g. electron microscopy) have been used in con-

Table 6
Immunochemical Studies on Membrane Proteins

Membrane Type	Organism or Tissue	Objectives	Antiserum to	Immunochemical measurements	Reference
Golgi apparatus	Rat liver	Characterization of Golgi enzymology	NADPH-cyto-chrome c reductase	Immunoinhibition titrations	Hino *et al.* (1978)
Golgi apparatus Microsomes Outer mitochondrial membrane	Rat liver	Demonstration of same enzymes in different membranes	NADH-cytochrome b_5 reductase cytochrome b_5	Immunoinhibition titrations double diffusion	Borgese and Meldolesi (1976)
Inner mitochondrial membrane	Yeast	Demonstration of site of synthesis of protein	cytochrome c_1	Immunoprecipitation	Ross and Schatz (1976)
	Yeast	Demonstration of site of synthesis of protein	cytochrome b	Immunoprecipitation	Lin *et al.* (1978)
	Yeast	Demonstration of site of synthesis of protein	cytochrome bc_1	Immunoprecipitation	Katan *et al.* (1976)
	Yeast	Demonstration of *in vitro* transcription and translation	cytochrome oxidase	Indirect Immunoprecipitation	Moorman *et al.* (1978)
Endoplasmic reticulum	Rat liver	Characterization of esterase enzymes	1. microsomes 2. inducible antigen	Rocket immunoelectrophoresis Zymogram staining Immunoinhibition titrations	Raftell *et al.* (1977)
	Rat liver	Enzyme topology	NAD-glyco-hydrolase	Immunoinhibition titrations	Bock and Matern (1973)
	Mouse liver	Delineation of haemoprotein involvement in drug metabolism	NADPH-cyto-chrome c reductase NADH-cyto-chrome b_5 reductase Cytochrome b_5	Double diffusion Immunoinhibition titrations	Noshiro and Omura (1978)

Source	Study	Enzyme system	Method	Reference
Pig liver (and others)	Participation of cytochrome P_{450} and amine oxidase in N-demethylation reactions	NADPH-cytochrome c reductase Microsomal amine oxidase	Immunoinhibition titrations	Pough and Ziegler (1977)
Rat liver	Characterization of multiplicity of cytochrome P_{450}	Cytochrome P_{450} Cytochrome P_{448}	Double diffusion Immunoinhibition titrations	Thomas et al. (1976)
Rat liver	Functional topology of cytochrome P_{450}	Cytochrome P_{450} Cytochrome P_{448}	Immunoinhibition titrations	Thomas et al. (1977)
Rat liver	Characterization of multiplicity of cytochrome P_{450}	Cytochrome P_{450} Cytochrome P_{448}	Double diffusion Immunoinhibition titrations	Ryan et al. (1977)
Rat liver	Characterization of enzyme heterogeneity in endoplasmic reticulum	Cytochrome b_5 (hybridized with antibodies to ferritin)	Electron microscopy	Remacle et al. (1976)
Rat liver	Delineation of mechanism of $\triangle 6$ desaturation	Cytochrome b_5	Immunoinhibition titrations	Lee et al. (1977)
Rat liver	Delineation of mechanism of oxidative detoxification	Cytochrome b_5 NADPH-cytochrome c reductase	Immunoinhibition titrations	Okayasu et al. (1977)
Rat liver	Identification of preneoplastic antigen	epoxide hydrase	Double diffusion	Levin et al. (1978)
Rat liver	Identification of enzyme(s) involved in hydration of polycyclic hydrocarbons	epoxide hydrase	Immunoinhibition titrations	Oesch and Bentley (1976)
Human erythrocytes	Identification of erythrocyte redox enzymes	NADH-cytochrome b_5 reductase cytochrome b_5	Immunoinhibition titrations	Kuma et al. (1976)

Membrane Type	Organism or Tissue	Objectives	Antiserum to	Immunochemical measurements	Reference
Sarcoplasmic reticulum	Rat	Accessibility of DNP groups covalently attached to sarcoplasmic ATP'ase	Dinitrophenol	Fluorescence Quenching Immunotitrations	Hardwicke (1976)
	Rat skeletal muscle cells	Measurement of enzyme synthetic rate	Adenosine triphosphatase	Immunoprecipitation	Holland and MacLennan (1976)
Plasma membrane	Erythrocytes	Immunochemical characterization of membrane	Erythrocyte membrane	Immunoelectrophoresis	Bjerrum and Bøg-Hansen (1976)
	Micrococcus luteus	Characterization of ATP'ase complex	F_1.ATP'ase	Crossed-Rocket immunoelectrophoresis	Schmitt et al. (1978)
	Rat liver and Ascites hepatoma AH-130	Characterization of membrane changes in tumour cells	Plasma membrane	Immunoinhibition titrations	Ikehara et al. (1977)
	Rat liver and hepatomas	Characterization of arylamidases in normal and transformed cells	Liver subcellular fractions	Immunoelectrophoresis with zymogram technique	Berzins et al. (1977a)
	Rat liver	Production of antisera to specific arylamidases	Zymogram identified esterase immunoprecipitates	Immunoelectrophoresis	Berzins et al. (1977b)
	Renal medulla	Separation of anti-catalytic and anti-ion transport antibodies	Na^+/K^+ ATP'ase	Immunoaffinity adsorption	McCans et al. (1974)
	Renal medulla	Study of species and tissue	i. ATP'ase catalytic site	Immunoinhibition titrations	McCans et al. (1975)

	Tissue	Purpose (differences in Na+/K+ ATP'ase)	Target (ii. ATP'ase ouabain receptor site)	Method	Reference
	Renal convoluted tubules	Localization of ATP'ase	Na$^+$/K$^+$ ATP'ase	Electron microscopy with ferritin conjugate	Kyte (1976)
	Electrophorus electroplax	Study of conformation and topology of ATP'ase	i. Large subunit of ATP'ase ii. holo-ATP'ase	Immunoinhibition Double diffusion Trypsin sensitivity of Immune Complex	Jean and Albers (1976)
Brush border	Pig intestine and kidney	Study of surface homology of aminopeptidases	Aminopeptidase	Immunoinhibition titrations	Louvard et al. (1976)
	intestine and kidney	Characterization of structural and topological homology of aminopeptidases	Aminopeptidase	Immunoinhibition titrations	Vannier et al. (1976)
	Intestine	To study orientation of aminopeptidase	Aminopeptidase	Macromolecular photolabelling	Louvard et al. (1976)
	Intestine	To study topological relationship of membrane proteins	Aminopeptidase sucrase	Agglutination	Takesue and Nishi (1976)
	Intestine	To study orientation of aminopeptidase in membrane	Aminopeptidase	Agglutination Electron microscopy	Takesue and Nishi (1978)
	Intestine and kidney	To study orientation of membrane vesicles	Aminopeptidase M	Immunoinhibition titrations	Haase et al. (1978)

junction with suitably modified antibodies (e.g. ferritin or peroxidase conjugated antibodies) in order to decide the location of a membrane enzyme. These methods can be used in parallel with methods which rely on the immunoinhibitory capacity of the antibodies (Chapter 4). Immunoinhibition has several problems, particularly related to incomplete inhibition at saturating concentrations of antibodies which can cause difficulties of interpretation. Precise location of antigens by immunochemical techniques linked to electron microscopy are also not without some problems of interpretation. However, immunochemical reagents have and will play a key role in defining membrane topography.

The precise location of membrane enzymes and proteins in cells must be known if the complex features of membrane biogenesis and degradation are to be understood. Therefore many workers wish to characterize the specific enzymology of some defined cellular membrane not only to understand the functions of the membrane but also to understand the interrelationships of its biogenesis with that of other cellular organelles (e.g. nuclear envelope and endoplasmic reticulum, outer mitochondrial membrane and endoplasmic reticulum). Antisera to specific enzymes and purified subcellular organelles have been used for these studies. The use of monospecific antisera is simpler than polyspecific antisera, in order to definitively ascribe an enzyme to some organelle, but a key to the use of either immunoreagent is the purity of the orginal membrane preparation. This is the classical problem of subcellular fractionation, namely how much contamination of some organelle preparations occurs. Marker enzymes have been routinely used to assess specific membrane enrichment during membrane purification and the degree of contamination by other cellular membranes. The results of extensive studies always indicate some degree of cross contamination. This poses potential problems immunochemically. Contamination of a membrane fraction used to raise a multispecific antiserum will obviously cause problems for immunoprecipitation analyses. These problems can be overcome to a large extent by adsorption of antisera with putative contaminating fractions. However, the use of a monospecific antiserum to a specific protein causes less difficulties when used as an immunoreagent for the characterization of specific membrane enzymology (see also Chapter 4).

Much attention in cell biology and biochemistry has been turned to problems of membrane biogenesis and membrane protein degradation. Immunochemical reagents to specific proteins provide the only reliable method for the rapid quantitative isolation of specific membrane proteins so that their rates of synthesis can be accurately estimated in normal physiological conditions or after experimental perturbation by pharmacological or other means. For example, antisera have played a key role in our present understanding of the biosynthetic interrelationships of mitochondrial proteins which have subunits which are synthesized on both mitochondrial and cytoplasmic polyribosomes. Recently, antisera to cytochrome oxidase have been used to identify protein sequences produced by the *in vitro* transcription and translation of mitochondrial DNA. Studies on membrane protein degradation can also be effectively carried out with antisera. Since our knowledge of protein degradation is so much less than that of protein synthesis the use of specific antisera to membrane proteins in combination with examination of the protein subunit(s) after isolation of the antigen (e.g. by polyacrylamide gel electrophoresis in the presence of sodium dodecyl sulphate) is the only way to unravel the complexities of membrane protein degradation.

It may be surprising, but many of the enzymological functions of cell membranes are currently not understood. The development of extensive studies on xenobiotic agents, particularly those which may be involved in chemical carcinogenesis, and the increasing development of new pharmacological agents has concentrated the efforts of many biomedical scientists on the complexities of the endoplasmic reticular drug detoxification system, particularly with respect to the inter-relationships of NADPH-cytochrome c reductase and NADH-cytochrome b_5 reductase in metabolism of xenobiotic substances. These studies have been carried out immunochemically and clearly indicate the usefulness of immunoreagents in the study of membrane enzymology.

The degree of microheterogeneity in the cellular membrane systems is a matter of conjecture and therefore of great interest. Morphological and therefore function heterogeneity of defined cellular membrane fractions is of particular interest. The interrelationships of endoplasmic reticulum, Golgi membranes, and plasma membranes as defined by their shared protein antigens is of key importance to the understanding of the endomembrane system and its biogenesis. Immunochemical reagents in combination with sophisticated centrifugation techniques can be used to define these relationships. Furthermore, immunochemical methods can be used to show whether membrane fragments obtained after membrane rupture and centrifugation (e.g. on continuous sucrose gradients) are related. This approach has been used to show that there is a heterogeneous distribution of proteins (e.g. cytochrome b_5) in the endoplasmic reticulum. This has been interpreted to mean that there are not specialized morphological and therefore functional regions of this membrane system.

Many immunochemical studies on membrane proteins have sought to establish the conformational homology of enzymes (e.g. Na$^+$/K$^+$ ATP$'$ase) in membranes from different tissues and different species. Immunochemical reagents can be extensively used in this type of work to define evolutionary conservation of structure and function.

Many membrane proteins have complex subunit structures. The functional and structural interactions of these subunits must be clearly defined if we are to understand the transport or enzymological role of these protein complexes. Several studies have been carried out where immunochemical reagents to the holoenzyme or holoprotein have been compared with immunoreagents generated to individual subunit(s) of a protein complex. Comparative use of these reagents gives information on the structural interactions of the components of the complex as well as information on functional interactions.

The conformational interrelationships of parts of the surfaces of membrane proteins can be examined conveniently by immunochemical reagents. The exposure of antigenic determinants can be used as a measure of conformational change in response to treatment of the protein with a variety of ligands. This approach is particularly useful in an attempt to describe which parts of proteins are exposed at a membrane surface and which parts are buried. This approach, when coupled with electron microscopy, has been used to estimate the extent to which membrane proteins protrude from the membrane surface.

The proximity of membrane proteins to each other has also been fruitfully investigated by immunochemical reagents. Two or more antibodies to specific proteins have been used to show the close interaction of the proteins in a membrane. The apposition of the different antigens has been deduced from studies where one immunoreagent (F_{ab} fragment) prevents access of another immunoreagent (whole antibody) to its antigen. This approach is particularly useful when membrane vesicle preparations can be prepared containing the antigens of interest, since the phenomenon of agglutination can be used as a tool to assess the closeness of heterologous antigens in a membrane.

If the vectorial orientation of a membrane antigen has been previously determined definitively (e.g. *in situ*) by an immunochemical or alternative technique, then an immunochemical reagent can be used to decide on the topology of membrane vesicles with respect to *in vivo* topology. An immunoreagent to a protein which has been shown to be on a particular side of a membrane can be used to determine whether vesicles (e.g. microvillus derived vesicles) are "right-side" or "inside" out. This is a prerequisite if such preparations are to be used for transport studies as is often the case.

Characterization of the membrane enzymology or protein profile by the immunochemical approaches described above can serve a further useful purpose, namely to define quantitatively the normal protein complement and protein distribution in a membrane. This profile can then be studied during cell transformation and tumorigenesis when the profile may significantly change, particularly in the plasma membrane of a cell. Polyspecific antisera to antigens in defined organelle fractions have been used to study these changes. Finally, in a related field, immunoreagents have proved useful in identifying precisely the nature of an enzyme which accumulates after insult of an experiment animal with proximate carcinogens or pharmacological agents. A typical problem is to show that an enzyme activity which increases in the endoplasmic reticulum in response to some treatment (e.g. with polycyclic hydrocarbons) is the same as a well-characterized endoplasmic reticulum enzyme. Alternatively, the functional or structural differences between an accumulating enzyme and a well-characterized enzyme must be assessed. Studies of this type have been carried out with epoxide hydrase and with cytochrome P_{450} polymorphs in response to a variety of xenobiotic agents.

By reading this summary of the immunochemical approaches used to study a variety of questions concerning membrane proteins it is clear that there is not a single property of these proteins which does not deserve an immunochemical study. The lists of specific immunochemical studies (Table 6) give the methodological detail and innovation of experimental design which has been adopted by scientists with diverse research interests in order to characterize the molecular biology of membrane proteins.

II. Immunochemical Studies on Membrane Proteins

A. Golgi Apparatus

The nature of the *in situ* enzymology of the Golgi apparatus is incompletely understood. A major problem concerns whether enzymes which are found in the Golgi apparatus and also in other membranes (particularly the endoplasmic reticulum) naturally occur in the Golgi apparatus or whether their presence is due to contamination of the Golgi apparatus with, for example, membrane from the endoplasmic reticulum. Resolution of this problem is important from the point of view of Golgi function and also with respect to Golgi biogenesis. Hino *et al.* (1978) have approached this problem with an antiserum to NADPH-cytochrome c reductase (a known endoplasmic reticulum enzyme). In order to study the nature of the Golgi enzyme they combined an immunochemical approach with the use of an aqueous polymer two-phase partition system which fractionates microsomes and Golgi apparatus. The Golgi enzyme is immunologically identical with the endoplasmic reticulum enzyme and is reported to occur on the cytoplasmic surface of the Golgi membranes since there is no change in the extent of immunoinhibition of the enzyme activity in the absence of presence of Triton X-100. Since the Golgi enzyme fractionates in the two-phase partition system in the same way as Golgi marker enzymes and not microsomal enzymes the authors conclude that NADPH-cytochrome c reductase is an *in vivo* constituent of Golgi membranes and is the same gene product (immunochemically) as in the endoplasmic reticulum. Biosynthetic implications (i.e. streaming of the enzyme to the Golgi from the endoplasmic reticulum) naturally follow from these observations.

It has been similarly shown that the NADH-cytochrome c reductase electron transport system of the endoplasmic reticulum, Golgi apparatus and mitochondrial outer membrane of rat liver is immunologically similar (Borgese and Meldolesi, 1976). The NADH-cytochrome c reductase activity is inhibited by approximately 80% in each membrane preparation by antisera to both NADH-cytochrome b_5 reductase and cytochrome b_5. The immunological identity of NADH-cytochrome b_5 reductase in microsomal and outer mitochondrial membranes has also been shown (Takesue and Omura, 1970).

B. *Inner Mitochondrial Membrane*

The bimodal sites of synthesis of mitochondrial membrane proteins have fascinated "mitochondriologists" for many years. Immunochemical methods alone have provided the means for ascribing a mitochondrial or cytoplasmic site of synthesis for some mitochondrial proteins. The immunological approach has been employed in conjugation with the use of drugs which inhibit mitoribosomal or cytoribosomal protein synthesis. Immunoprecipitation of detergent-solubilized mitochondria has often been the method of choice, combined with separation of the subunit(s) of the immunoisolated proteins by polyacrylamide gel electrophoresis in the presence of sodium dodecyl sulphate. Problems of non-specific precipitation may be encountered due to the extreme hydrophobicity of the membrane proteins. This requires careful controls with non-immune serum instead of antiserum. Several of the problems associated with non-specific precipitation may be overcome by the use of immunoaffinity chromotography (Chapter 4).

The conclusions of these investigations are that cytochrome c_1 is synthesized on cytoplasmic ribosomes (Ross and Schatz, 1976); cytochrome b is synthesized on mitochondrial ribosomes; and that of the seven polypeptides of the cytochrome bc_1 complex only one is synthesized on mitochondrial ribosomes and that, as expected, is cytochrome b (Katan *et al.*, 1976).

Yeast mitochondrial DNA has been transcribed and translated in an *E.coli* cell free system to give protein products in which some cytochrome oxidase sequences can be identified by indirect immunoprecipitation (Moorman *et al.*, 1978). The cytochrome oxidase sequences were shown to be incomplete. They were identified after immunoprecipitation by poly-acrylamide gel electrophoresis in the presence of sodium dodecyl sulphate. Their identity as cytochrome oxidase sequences was supported by immuno-competition studies with pure yeast cytochrome oxidase. The presence of cytochrome oxidase sequences was confirmed with antisera to the holo-enzyme and with antisera to subunits (I + II) and subunit II. The authors comment on the specificity of the antisera (which may also react to some extent with components of the cytochrome bc_1 complex) and suggest that antibody specificity should be determined under conditions which resemble as nearly as possible those pertaining in product identification. This is a pertinent observation for all those engaged in studies with antisera to membrane proteins and is to be recommended even when antibody populations purified by immunoaffinity chromatography (Chapter 4) are used. Essentially, the subunit composition of an antigen of interest must be known and immunoisolated products should be analysed and shown to only contain subunits to the antigen of interest. Naturally problems will arise when putative contaminants have similar subunit sizes to subunits of the antigen of interest.

C. Endoplasmic Reticulum

Many immunochemical studies with diverse objectives have been carried out on microsomal proteins, particularly haem proteins. Specific examples to illustrate the diversity of approaches taken in various studies are given in Table 6.

Raftell *et al.* (1977) have investigated microsomal esterase activities, specifically the phenobarbital-inducible esterase in rat liver. The approach is typical of that carried out in several membrane protein studies where a multispecific antiserum (i.e. to microsomal proteins) is first used in combination with crossed-rocket immunoelectrophoresis and a zymogram technique. Esterase multiplicity is demonstrated by this approach and a specific esterase immunoprecipitate identified which increased in proportion relative to the other precipitates in zymograms of microsomal preparations taken from phenobarbital treated animals. This immunoprecipitate was used to prepare a monospecific antiserum which was used to inspect tissue distribution and membrane sideness of this drug inducible antigen. The use of immunoprecipitates to raise monospecific antisera and the problems of the method are discussed later. However, the approach is very useful in providing antisera to proteins which otherwise would be very difficult to obtain.

Purification of microsomal proteins after solubilization with proteolytic enzymes is commonly used to obtain the "hydrophilic" portions of integral membrane proteins. The solubilized preparations are then used for antiserum production. This approach has been very successfully employed for haem proteins as discussed below. Another novel approach has been used in the purification of NAD-glycohydrolase from microsomes (Bock and Matern, 1973) where porcine pancreatic lipase was used to solubilize the enzyme. However, it may be that this lipase preparation was contaminated with proteolytic enzymes. The antiserum raised to this preparation immunoinhibited 60–80% of the activity of the "lipase-solubilized" enzyme but only 20–30% of the enzyme activity *in situ* in the microsomal membrane and in Triton X–100 microsomal extracts. The authors interpreted the limited accessibility to antibodies *in situ* as indicating buried enzyme or the fact that the enzyme was located inside the microsomal vesicles.

Many authors have used antisera, sometimes in combination with other techniques (e.g. proteolytic removal of antigens from a membrane) to determine the vectorial orientation of antigens. In microsomal studies this objective has been achieved along with the main objectives which have been the elucidation of the pathways of electron transport and the roles of the known haem protein complexes in the oxidation of drugs. The immunoinhibition of drug oxidations by antisera has been used as a criterion for the involvement of the specific antigen in the oxidation process. This elegant use of immunoinhibition in the delineation of metabolic processes in microsomes has been perfected in studies reported by Noshiro and Omura (1978). Here immunoaffinity purified antibodies to NADPH-cytochrome c reductase, NADH-cytochrome b_5 reductase, cytochrome b_5 and cytochrome P_{450} were used to immunobinhibit their respective antigens. Through a combination of the use of antisera and antigen removal by trypsinization the authors showed that NADPH-cytochrome c reductase is an essential component in electron flow to cytochrome P_{450} for most drug oxidations, whereas NADH-cytochrome b_5 reductase and cytochrome b_5 participate in NADH supported oxidation of some but not all drugs.

These authors were fortunate in that large immunoinhibitions of microsomal oxidations were achieved with the respective antisera. This is essential for simple interpretation of results and contrasts with studies reported on NADH-glycohydrolase (Bock and Matern, 1973) and monoamine oxidase (Russell *et al.*, 1978b). The studies of Noshiro and Omura (1978) on immunoinhibition of drug oxidation are extremely elegant allowing a proposal of a schematic representation of electron transport pathways in the microsomal electron transfer system. The specificity of antisera provides a tool for the inspection of metabolic processes which cannot be achieved readily by any other means. The use of immunoinhibition of a process as criterion of antigen involvement in a metabolic process will be of less value when little immunoinhibition takes place. This is the only restriction in the use of the approach. Antisera to cytochrome b_5 and NADPH-cytochrome c reductase have been used to delineate the mechanism of microsomal 6-desaturation of fatty acids. The results of immunoinhibition titrations provide clear evidence that a cytochrome b_5 linked process is involved (Lee et al., 1977) and that NADPH-cytochrome c reductase is not involved (Okayasu et al., 1977). Both these studies were again dependent on the large immunoinhibition of fatty acid desaturation by the respective antisera.

Prough and Ziegler (1977) have similarly used the immunoinhibition criterion to show that NADPH-cytochrome c (P_{450}) reductase is partly involved in N-demethylation reactions in microsomes. However, further delineation of the process by a similar approach with antibodies to purified microsomal amine oxidase was prevented by the lack of immunoinhibitory capacity of this antiserum.

Growing interest in the effect of xenobiotic agents, particularly putative proximate carcinogens, on the endoplasmic reticulum, has led to further detailed studies on the liver microsomal electron transport system. Antisera to cytochrome P_{450} (prepared from phenobarbital-treated rats) have been used to study the multiplicity of cytochrome P_{450} (Thomas et al., 1976; Thomas et al., 1977). These studies indicate that at least six different forms of immunochemically related species of cytochrome P_{450} could be detected. Immunochemically cytochrome P_{450} and cytochrome P_{448} are also partially related. Immunoinhibition titrations confirm a multiplicity of cytochromes P_{450}. Whether the multiple forms are derived from a single gene product is not clear from these studies. Further work has indicated a marked difference in the proportions of the different forms of cytochrome P_{450} in microsomes from phenobarbital, methylcholanthrene and pregnenolone-16-carbonitrile treated rats (Thomas et al., 1977). Antiserum was also used here to show that cytochrome P_{450} is at least partially exposed to the hydrophilic environment on the exterior of microsomal membranes. The antisera to cytochrome P_{450} and cytochrome P_{448} were similarly used to show that the increased production of cytochromes in response to the polychlorinated biphenyl mixture, Araclor 1254, is very similar to that induced by phenobarbital (Ryan et al., 1977).

This approach could be usefully extended to examine the complexities of the changes in the endoplasmic reticulum oxidative enzymology in response to specific carcinogens in order to determine the involvement of the different electron transport systems in the oxidative metabolism of these compounds.

The further metabolism of oxidized carcinogens may be carried out by epoxide hydrase. This enzyme was originally assayed with styrene oxide as substrate and it was therefore of interest to know whether the same enzyme was involved in the hydration of benz(a)pyrene 4,5 oxide and other epoxides derived from carcinogenic polycyclic hydrocarbons. Antibodies to purified epoxide hydrase have been successfully used in immunoinhibition titrations to show that there is a single enzyme species which hydrates styrene oxide and benz(a)pyrene 4,5 oxide (Oesch and Bentley, 1976).

More recently, antibodies to epoxide hydrase have been used to show that a prenloplastic antigen found in 2-acetylamino fluorene induced hyperplastic nodules in liver is immunochemically identical with epoxide hydrase. The enzyme is present in the nodules at five times the concentration found in surrounding non-tumour tissue (Levin *et al.*, 1978).

The studies with monospecific antisera to microsomal antigens clearly indicated the value of antisera in elucidating biochemical pathways involved in drug metabolism and particularly in the characterization of the response of liver endoplasmic reticulum to xenobiotic putative carcinogenic agents.

D. *Sarcoplasmic Reticulum*

Several immunochemical studies on sarcoplasmic reticulum adenosine triphosphatase (ATP'ase) have been carried out. A novel approach has been to use anti-dinitrophenol antibodies to detect the number of accessible dinitrophenylated moieties attached to sulphydryl groups in the ATP'ase of sarcoplasmic vesicles (Hardwicke, 1976). The sulphydryl groups were modified by reaction with 1-(2,4-dinitrophenylamino,6-(*N*-maleimido)hexane or N_1N'-bis(2,4-dinitrophenyl)-L-cystine. Fluorescence quenching titrations of anti-dinitrophenyl-antibody tryptophyl fluorescence of the dinitrophenyl-vesicle conjugates was measured. The results were interpreted to mean that not all the dinitrophenyl groups were accessible to the antibody.

It is interesting to speculate that this approach of probing a functional enzyme site by means of antibodies to a modifying agent of some functional group may be more generally applicable. This would be of great value if the technique could be applied with antibodies to ligands which act non-covalently at the functional site(s) of a protein. For example, it may be possible to probe neurotransmitter receptors by the combined use of agonists or antagonists and antibodies to these pharmacological agents. This would only be practicable if the "off-rate" of the ligands was very slow.

Antibodies to the ATP'ase have also been used to study the rate of synthesis of the enzyme in rat skeletal muscle cells in tissue culture. This type of study helps to clarify the cell biological events occurring during myogenesis (Holland and MacLennan, 1976).

E. Plasma Membrane

Plasma membrane antigens have been and are the subject of innumerable studies in many fields of biomedicine, particularly in immunology and cancer research and are therefore out of the scope of this book. However, the diversity of uses of immunochemical methods in studying plasma membrane proteins are shown in Table 6.

Immunoelectrophoresis with multispecific or monospecific antisera has been widely used to study protein topology in plasma membranes. The general problems in studying membrane proteins have been stressed throughout the book but this is a good opportunity to point out that immunoprecipitation techniques, which have been extensively used for plasma membrane antigens, can be significantly influenced by protease or glycosidase modification of antigens and that careful choice of detergent (i.e. non-ionic) is required to avoid other possible antigen alterations. With attention to these points good immunochemical analysis of membrane protein antigens by immunoprecipitation techniques in agarose gels can be carried out (Bjerrum and Bøg-Hansen, 1976b).

Multispecific antisera to plasma membranes (Ikehara et al., 1977) or subcellular membranes including plasma membranes (Berzins et al., 1977) have been used to study alkaline phosphatase, 5'-nucleotidase and arylamidase. From a combined use of lectin inhibition and immunoinhibition titrations Ikehara et al. (1977) conclude that 50% of the 5'-nucleotidase activity of plasma membrane was not due to activity of 5'-nucleotidase but to alkaline phosphatase which also hydrolyses 5'-AMP.

Fused rocket immunoelectrophoresis has been used to show the presence of arylamidase antigens (identified by staining the rockets, i.e. the zymogram technique), in plasma membranes, lysosomes and microsomes (Berzins et al., 1977a). In general this approach may suffer from the fact that it is probably impossible to obtain subcellular organelles free from cross contamination and therefore this may make the use of multispecific antisera prepared from these fractions difficult to interpret.

Berzins et al. (1977b) have tried to prepare monospecific antisera against the microsomal and lysosomal arylamidases by immunization with im-

munoprecipitate lines obtained from crossed-rocket immunoelectrophoresis carried out with the polyspecific antisera. The work highlights
some of the difficulties, since two cycles of immunization and crossed-
rocket immunoelectrophoresis were needed to obtain monospecific antiserum to the microsomal arylamidase, while three cycles of immunization
were needed to obtain monospecific antiserum to the lysosomal arylamidase (Berzins *et al.*, 1977b). This serves to show that immunoprecipitates,
which do not strain for a particular enzyme activity can occur with the
staining antigen–antibody precipitate and can therefore be injected along
with the antigen of interest during an attempt to produce a monospecific
antiserum.

There is much interest in the Na^+/K^+ ATP'ase of plasma membranes in
many tissues and organisms particularly in relation to its role in ion
transport. The ATP'ase in the plasma membrane of *Micrococcus luteus* can
be operationally divided into an easily released part (i.e. released by
osmotic shock) called the F_1.ATP'ase which is associated in the membrane
in the so-called F_0.F_1 ATP'ase complex. This is released from the
membrane by Triton X-100. Immunoaffinity purified antibodies to the
F_1.ATP'ase completely inhibits the F_0.F_1 ATP'ase and crossed immunoelectrophoresis reveals a complete reaction of identity between the
F_1.ATP'ase and the Triton X-100 solubilized F_1.F_0 ATP'ase indicating that
both enzymes have common antigenic sites (Schmitt *et al.*, 1978). This
approach shows the value of an immunochemical method to show the
relationship between an easily derived moiety of a membrane protein
complex and the parent complex in the plasma membrane.

A more sophisticated immunochemical approach to the Na^+/K^+
ATP'ase has been adopted for the renal medulla by McCans *et al.* (1974,
1975). In these studies immunoaffinity purified antibodies to the holoenzyme were fractionated with the ouabain-holoenzyme complex into a
binding anti-catalytic antibody fraction and a non-binding anti-cardiac
glycoside binding fraction. The anti-catalytic antibodies were dissosiated
from the immunoprecipitate by acid treatment and used along with the
anti-glycoside binding site antibodies to study the properties of the
enzyme isolated from different organs and species. Such an approach
provides antibodies which can define the different functional regions of the
membrane ATP'ase. The antibodies can also be used as conformation-
detecting probes when the enzyme reacts with its substrates.

An alternative approach to the study of the Na^+/K^+ ATP'ase has been
taken with the enzyme from *Electrophorus* electroplax organ. Here the
effects of an antiserum to the 96 000 mol. wt large subunit was compared
with an antiserum to the holoenzyme (Jean and Albers, 1976). The
antiserum to the large enzyme subunit inhibits ATP'ase activity and

enzyme phosphorylation. The K^+-sensitive dephosphorylation was un-changed. The antiserum to the holoenzyme produced similar effects. These authors studied the effects of trypsin on the immune complexes obtained with the Lubrol solubilized enzyme and the antiserum to the large subunit and the holoenzyme. The results show that the antiholoenzyme protects the whole molecule from trypsin while the anti-large subunit protects only the large subunit. This experiment was interpreted to mean that the large and small subunits of the ATP'ase are well separated (in view of the size of the immunoglobulin molecule) and could be on different sides of the membrane *in vivo*. Here again antisera are judiciously used to probe the conformation and topography of a membrane enzyme.

F. Brush Border

Several elegant studies have been carried out by immunochemical methods on the topology of proteins in the microvillus membrane of the brush border of enterocytes and kidney proximal tubules. These studies are exemplory in that they show the great value of immunochemical studies on membrane proteins when the phenomena are interpreted in terms of the molecular interactions of antibodies with a macromolecular antigen. Louvard *et al.* (1976a, b) have proposed that a protein antigen, when used as immunogen, will stimulate the production of antibodies directed specifi-cally against the exposed determinants on its surface. The maximum number of antibody molecules that can bind simultaneously to the antigen corresponds, therefore, to the complete covering of the macromolecular surface. If the molecular weight of the protein is known together with that of the immunoglobulin then the maximum antibody binding can be expressed in terms of moles of antibody per mole of antigen. When immunotitrations are carried out with iodinated immunoaffinity-purified antibodies at either fixed antigen or fixed antibody concentration the extent of saturation of antigenic determinants can be measured. If a fixed concentration of antibody is used with increasing concentrations of anti-gen, the graph of unbound radioactivity (i.e. in the antibody) versus the antibody/antigen ratio will be as shown in Fig. 36. The extrapolated value is taken as the antibody/antigen ratio corresponding to complete covering of the antigen surface with antibody and is therefore a measure of the number of determinants exposed on the surface of the protein.

The number of exposed determinants is very useful in the study of membrane proteins since it may vary when the same protein is present in different membranes (e.g. intestinal and kidney brush border). The number of exposed determinants will give a measure of the degree of exposure of the antigen in the membrane. Naturally the number of

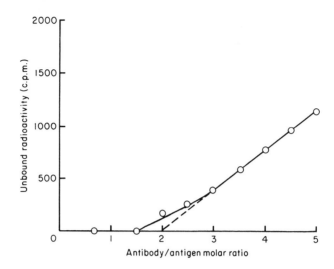

Fig. 36. Saturation of antigenic sites on proteins. Increasing amounts (moles) of antigen are added to a fixed amount (mole) of radiolabelled (iodinated) antibody (or F_{ab} fragment). The radioactivity which is not precipitated or which can be separated from F_{ab}-Antigen by gel filtration is plotted versus the antibody/antigen molar ratio. The extrapolated line gives a measure of the number of antigenic determinants on the surface of the protein.

determinants can also be estimated in solubilized preparations of the antigen. A potential problem with this method must be that of steric hindrance whereby binding of antibody to the surface of a protein may prevent further binding of antibodies to other antigenic determinants on the protein surface. This problem may be overcome to some degree by the use of F_{ab} fragments derived from the antibodies of interest (Louvard et al., 1976b).

With this method it has been shown that aminopeptidases in the pig intestinal and kidney brush border membrane have six identical antigenic determinants, two of which are located in the area that is masked upon integration of the enzyme into the membrane.

Further studies have been carried out with the free (detergent or trypsin solubilized) form of the aminopeptidase and the membrane bound (vesicular) form derived from intestinal or renal brush borders (Vannier et al., 1976). The antibodies used were prepared against the renal enzyme and adsorbed by immunoaffinity chromatography with the intestinal enzyme linked to Sepharose. The eluate (57% of the total antibodies) was considered to contain antibodies to common antigenic determinants on both the renal and intestinal enzymes. The results of the subsequent immunotitrations were interpreted to mean that the enzymes from the two sites contained six cross-reacting determinants. This is consistent with a high degree of structural homology. Four of these determinants were accessible in the bound form of the enzymes. The other two determinants were completely masked in the bound form and may therefore be associated with the junction between the hydrophilic and hydrophobic moieties of the membrane enzyme. The authors proposed that since most crystallographic data suggest that mutations of globular proteins affect surface residues the use of the this type of immunochemical technique, which explores the antigen surface, is excellent to probe interspecies structural homology in proteins.

Vesicular preparations of the brush border were used in these studies of the aminopeptidase. These preparations are of great value for simplifying immunochemical studies (cf. *in situ* studies) and are, naturally, of great value for transport work, particularly since the brush border membrane vesiculates "right-side" out (see later). These vesicular preparations have been used to immunochemically study another problem concerning the aminopeptidase, namely, whether it is a transmembranous protein (Louvard *et al.*, 1976b). This immunochemical approach is very sophisticated and deserves mention in some detail so that other potential uses of the approach in different membrane systems could be considered.

In order to show that the enzyme was exposed on the inner face of the vesicular membrane, as well as the outer face, a photosensitive reagent was attached to the F_{ab} fragment of human myeloma protein and incorporated in the dark into the "right-side" out vesicles prepared from the enterocyte brush border. The reagent was 4-fluoro-3-nitrophenylazide, which when photolysed produces a nitrene capable of reacting with a variety of chemical bonds including those in proteins. Therefore photolysis of the vesiculated myeloma protein-reagent results in binding of the myeloma protein to moieties facing the inside of the vesicle including the proteins. The brush border vesicles are solubilized in detergent and the aminopeptidase is recognized and precipitated by the specific antibody. The elegance of attaching the reagent to the F_{ab} fragment of myeloma protein is that the extent of labelling of the aminopeptidase can be estimated by the reaction of the F_{ab} fragment of the myeloma protein with a monovalent anti-F_{ab} labelled with peroxidase.

By this approach aminopeptidase was shown to be a transmembraneous protein which is exposed at the inner and outer surface of the vesicles. Furthermore the labelling of the inward facing portion of the enzyme was in a hydrophobic region tightly associated with the membrane. Three regions of the aminopeptidase were proposed, a major region on the outer surface of the membrane, a hydrophobic part embedded within the phospholipid bilayer, and an inward facing region.

The usefulness of this type of immunochemical approach may be limited by the ease of production of vesicular preparations. Perhaps more difficulties will be found in meeting the requirement of minimizing non-specificity of the light-activated reagent upon which interpretation of the data depends.

An alternative principle has been used to study proteins in microvilli vesicles (Takesue and Nishi, 1976). Here the phenomenon of agglutination, as induced immunochemically, has been exploited to study the proximity of two antigens exposed on the outer surface of brush border vesicles. Agglutination is assayed by measuring the activities of microvillus enzymes and their sedimentation after antibody treatment) by low speed centrifugation. The assumption of the method is that if two antigens (A and B) are in close proximity on the membrane, then agglutination of the vesicles by Anti-A antiserum will be prevented by monovalent fragments (F_{ab}) of Anti-B antiserum (and *vice versa*). This approach has been carried out with microvillus vesicles and antisera to sucrase-isomaltase and aminopeptidase. Both antisera agglutinate the vesicles and F_{ab} fragments of each antibody population prevents agglutination by the other antibody population. However, the immunoinhibitory capacity of each antibody population in the presence of F_{ab} to the other antigen is not impaired. The authors conclude that sucrase-isomaltase and aminopeptidase are in close proximity on the outer surface of the vesicular membrane. In a further study by the combined use of agglutination, immunoinhibition and electron microscopy the authors concluded that the aminopeptidase protrudes some 10 nm above the outer surface of the vesicular membrane. Clearly agglutination of vesicle preparations has great scope for the study of the interrelationships between the mosaic of proteins which face outside in the plasma membrane of cells.

Finally, although not discussed when describing the immunochemical methods above, immunochemical techniques can be used to decide on the orientation of vesicular preparations prepared from cell membranes. Naturally this requires knowledge (perhaps derived immunochemically) of the *in situ* orientation of an antigen in the unperturbed membrane. With this knowledge a variety of techniques particularly immunoinhibition titration or agglutination can be used to show the proportion of vesicles which are "right-side" out or "inside" out.

This approach has been used by Haase *et al.* (1978) who used immunoinhibition titrations to show that brush border vesicles prepared from intestinal or kidney preparations are predominantly (perhaps greater than 90%) "right-side" out. The importance of this fact for transport studies cannot be overestimated.

In the future the use of antibodies to study membrane proteins can only increase. Without doubt antibodies are excellent reagents for use as membrane impermeable probes. As mentioned frequently in this book the specific methods used must depend on the particular antigen–antibody system of interest. Some particular or peculiar property of a membrane antigen could be exploited in order to fashion an immunoassay system. As elsewhere in biomedical science the use of more than one approach reduces difficulties of interpretation. More than one immunochemical method should be attempted when studying a membrane antigen.

6

Case Study II: Antigens in the Nervous System

I. Introduction

The brain, as the most complex of the tissues, is one of the most challenging of all biological systems to study since out of its physical complexity emerges that strange metaphysical entity, the mind. The complexity of the brain makes it difficult to know how one can ever understand how it works and it would be foolish to suggest that the mystery of the mind can be solved simply by applying immunochemical techniques to the study of the brain. However, one great advantage of antisera is that they can be used as biochemical, morphological and behaviour-modifying tools. Thus biochemically, antisera may be used to study the mechanism of synaptic transmission in terms of the presynaptic synthesis, degradation, storage and release of transmitter, and in terms of the postsynaptic effect of released transmitter. Morphologically, antisera may be used to determine the subcellular localization of an antigen, which type of cell it is associated with, and to trace neural pathways for specific transmitters (e.g. Table 7). Finally antisera may be used to induce behavioural changes in experimental animals (Hyden, 1973; Williams and Schupf, 1977).

In general two approaches have been attempted in immunochemical studies on the brain. In the first approach, a polyspecific antiserum is produced to the whole brain, cerebellum, etc. or to a subcellular fraction and then specific antigens are identified and characterized, if possible, by means of monospecific antisera. In the second approach monospecific antisera are prepared to individual components of known function or subcellular localization. In Table 8 a group of antigens associated with the nervous system are listed. Antigens of the cholinergic and adrenergic

Table 7
Immunocytochemically localized hormones and neuroactive peptides

Antigen	Reference
Adrenocorticotrophin	Watson et al., 1978
Enkephalin	Schultzberg et al., 1978
	Schultzberg et al., 1979
	Uhl et al., 1979
GABA	Saito, 1978
Gonadotropin releasing hormone	McNeill and Sladek, 1978
α-Melanocyte stimulating hormone	Swaab and Fisser, 1977
Non-peptide morphine-like compounds	Gintzler et al., 1978
Precursor of corticotropin, endorphin and melanotropin	Loh, 1979
Prolactin	Fuxe et al., 1977
Somatostatin	Hokfelt et al., 1975
	Schultzberg et al., 1978
Substance P	Fuxe et al., 1977
	Schultzberg et al., 1978

systems of synaptic transmission will be considered in detail and emphasis will be placed on phenomena of general relevance to biological scientists interested in immunochemical studies on specific antigens.

II. Antigens in the Cholinergic Synapse

In a system as complex as the brain it is difficult to study any one system of synaptic transmission in isolation since preparations of synaptosomes and synaptic vesicles are always heterogeneous with regard to transmitter and are often heavily contaminated with other subcellular fractions. For this reason the purely cholinergic electric organs of electric fish such as *Electrophorus* and *Torpedo* have become widely used for studies on the molecular mechanisms by which acetylcholine is synthesized, stored and degraded (Whittaker, 1977) and for studies on the postsynaptic effect of released acetylcholine (Heidmann and Changeux, 1978). Three of the most important proteins associated with the metabolism and function of acetylcholine are choline acetyltransferase, acetylcholinesterase and the acetylcholine receptor. These proteins have been studied extensively and may be discussed at length.

Table 8
Antigens in the Nervous System

Class	Tissue localization	Subcellular location	Function	Subunit molecular weight	References
Adrenergic Antigens					
Chromogranin A	Adrenal medulla Sympathetic nerves	Soluble vesicle protein	—	74–81 000	Winkler *et al.*, 1974 Lagercrantz, 1976 Winkler *et al.*, 1974
Chromomembrin B	Adrenal medulla Sympathetic nerves	Membrane protein	Unknown	27–28 000	Winkler *et al.*, 1974 Lagercrantz, 1976 Winkler *et al.*, 1974
Tyrosine hydroxylase	Adrenal medulla Sympathetic nerves	Cytoplasm	Synthesis of DOPA	34 000	Nagatsu and Kondo, 1975; Pickel *et al.*, 1975; Hoeldtke and Kaufman, 1977
DOPA decarboxylase	Adrenal medulla Sympathetic nerves	Cytoplasm	Synthesis of dopamine	110 000	Hökfelt *et al.*, 1973
Dopamine β hydroxylase	Adrenal medulla Sympathetic nerves	Vesicle protein	Synthesis of noradrenalin	75 000	Winkler, 1976; Helle *et al.*, 1979
Phenylethanolamine N-methyltransferase	Adrenal medulla Sympathetic nerves	Cytoplasm	Synthesis of adrenalin	40 000	Hökfelt *et al.*, 1973; Hökfelt *et al.*, 1974
Cholinergic Antigens					
Acetylcholinesterase	Neuromuscular	Membrane protein	Hydrolysis of acetylcholine (ACh)	76–80 000	Rieger *et al.*, 1976; Anglister *et al.*, 1979
Acetylcholine receptor	Neuromuscular	Membrane protein	Binds ACh; causes depolarisation	45 000; 50 000; 60 000; 65 000 (Torpedo)	Karlin *et al.*, 1978
Choline acetyl transferase	Motor neurones	Presynaptic cytoplasm	Synthesis of ACh	60–65 000	Heidmann and Changeux, 1978 Rossier, 1975; Kan *et al.*, 1978

Filamentous Antigens				
Actin	Ubiquitous	Motility	45 000	Lazarides, 1976; Blomberg et al., 1977
Myosin	Ubiquitous	Motility	200 000	Roisen et al., 1978; Unsicker et al., 1978
Microtubules	Ubiquitous	Structural	>300 000; 55 000; 54 000	Morgan et al., 1977
10 nm filaments e.g. desmin, e.g. neurofilament protein	Ubiquitous	Structural	55–55 000	Jorgensen et al., 1976; Schlaepfer, 1977; Gilbert, 1978; Lazarides and Hubbard 1978
Glial fibrillary acidic protein	Glia	Unknown	47 000	Zomzely–Neurath and Keller, 1977; Bocke, 1978
Nerve Specific Antigens				
S–100	Glia	Unknown	≃7000	Zomzely–Neurath and Keller, 1977; Bock, 1978
14-3-2	Neuronal	Enolase	48 000	Zomzely–Neurath and Keller, 1977; Bock, 1978
Synaptin	Membrane protein	Unknown	45 000	Zomzely–Neurath and Keller, 1977; Bock, 1978
D2	Membrane protein	Unknown	139 000	Zomzely–Neurath and Keller, 1977; Bock, 1978
D3	Membrane protein	Unknown	14–50 000	Zomzely–Neurath and Keller, 1977; Bock, 1978
D400	Cerebellum	Unknown	400 000	Zomzely–Neurath and Keller, 1977; Bock, 1978
Glutamate decarboxylase	Neuronal	Synthesis of GABA	85 000	McLaughlin et al., 1975
Tryptophan hydroxylase	Neuronal	Synthesis of serotonin		Reis et al., 1975

A. Choline Acetyltransferase

The purification of an antigen to homogeneity by biochemical criteria is usually an essential prerequisite to the production of a monospecific antiserum. In the case of choline acetyltransferase there is some controversy over the purity of preparations which have been used for the production of antisera (Rossier, 1975; Chao *et al.*, 1977). Thus the highest specific activities described for the enzyme are 25–30 μmol of acetycholine synthesized min^{-1} mg^{-1} protein (11 900 fold purification) from the caudate nucleus of bovine brain (Malthe-Sørenssen *et al.*, 1978); 20 μmol min^{-1} mg^{-1} (30 000 fold) from rat brain (Rossier, 1976a), and 30 μmol min^{-1} mg^{-1} (8570 fold) from the electric organ of *Torpedo californica* (Brandon and Wu, 1978). With the possible exception of the enzyme from *Torpedo* it seems likely that the final preparations contain contaminating proteins and that the purified enzyme exists as a single polypeptide of molecular weight 63–69 000. An interesting immunochemical approach to the purification of the enzyme has also been used (Malthe-Sørenssen *et al.*, 1973; Rossier, 1976a). Thus, after raising antisera to the partially purified antigen and finding no cross-reactivity with choline acetyltransferase these workers prepared immunoadsorbents through which they passed their partially purified enzyme preparations. This procedure removed the contaminating proteins to which the antisera had been raised. In both cases the immunoadsorbents were prepared by coupling IgG to cyanogen bromide activated Sepharose.

Antisera have been raised to choline acetyltransferase purified from several sources (Eng *et al.*, 1974; Shuster and O'Toole, 1974; Singh and McGeer, 1974; Rossier, 1976b; Malthe-Sørenssen *et al.*, 1978) and have been characterized by immunoprecipitation tests in agarose gels and by immunoprecipitation of enzyme activity. In some cases a single immunoprecipitation line was detected by immunodiffusion studies (Eng *et al.*, 1974; Singh and McGreer, 1974) and the enzyme was inactivated by incubation with the antiserum. These authors concluded, therefore, that they had obtained monospecific antisera to choline acetyltransferase and this may in fact be the case. However, it is also possible that although antibodies to choline acetyltransferase are present in the serum, they do not result in the formation of a visible immunoprecipitate on immunodiffusion. Indeed it is always essential to demonstrate that an immunoprecipitate contains the antigen of interest. Thus these authors should have cut out the immunoprecipitate formed on immunodiffusion and shown that it contained choline acetyltransferase activity. Alternatively, they could have used the antiserum to precipitate enzyme from radioactively labelled extracts and then analysed the immunprecipitates by polyacrylamide gel electrophoresis in the presence of sodium dodecyl sulphate in order to identify the enzyme subunit. Only a demonstration such as this will conclusively show that a monospecific antiserum to choline acetyltransferase has in fact been obtained. In cases where polyspecific antisera have been obtained, and choline acetyltransferase can be found to correspond to a specific immunoprecipitate, the immunoprecipitate may be used to immunize new animals to produce a monospecific antiserum (Koch and Nielsen, 1975).

The discussion above makes it difficult to assess some of the results obtained with antisera to choline acetyltransferase. Most of the groups who have raised antisera have done so with the intention of localizing cholinergic neurones and pathways in the central nervous system. The work on the immunohistochemical localization of choline acetyltransferase has been strongly criticized (Rossier, 1975). However, it is clear that the antisera used do contain antibodies to choline acetyltranferase (Shuster and O'Toole, 1974; Singh and McGeer, 1974; Chao et al., 1977) and, furthermore, positive immunochemical staining does seem to occur with cells which are known to be cholinergic by microdissection and microenzymatic analysis (Chao et al., 1977; Kan et al., 1978). Thus the peroxidase-antiperoxidase immunohistochemical method (Sternberger et al., 1970) has been used to localize antigen in formalin-fixed, paraffin-embedded sections of rabbit spinal cord and cerebellum (Kan et al., 1978). In the spinal cord the cell bodies of ventral horn motor neurones were labelled and in the cerebellum the antigen was localized in the mossy fibres and the glomeruli of the cerebella folia. Thus in this case at least it may be that the antigen localized is indeed choline acetyltransferase. However, until it is clearly demonstrated that these antisera are monospecific, all work on the immunohistochemical localization of choline acetyltransferase must be viewed with caution.

One fact which has been established with antisera to this enzyme is the strong evolutionary conservation of the choline acetyltransferase molecule. The antisera raised by Rossier (1976b) to the enzyme purified from rat brain was found to cross-react with choline acetyltransferase in crude extracts of chick brain and *Torpedo* electric organ. Similarly an antiserum prepared to choline acetyltransferase from bovine brain (Malthe-Sørenssen et al., 1978) cross-reacted with the enzyme from several other mammalian species. This demonstrates one great advantage of immunochemical techniques; that it is often possible to study a specific antigen in a tissue of interest with an antiserum prepared to an antigen from a different species for which a well-characterized purification procedure is available.

An antiserum to choline acetyltransferase from rat brain has been used to demonstrate that the decrease in choline acetyltransferase in cholinergic hypoglossal neurones after lesion of the hypoglossal nerve is in fact due to a decrease in the amount of enzyme protein (Wooten *et al.*, 1978). It was shown by immunotitration that the same amount of antiserum was required to precipitate a fixed amount of enzyme activity before and after lesion of the nerve. This method possesses the great advantage that a monospecific antiserum is not required.

B. *Acetylcholinesterase*

Acetylcholinesterase exists in a variety of molecular forms and the most complete characterization of these forms has come from studies on the enzyme purified from the electric organs of *Electrophorus* and *Torpedo marmorata* (Rieger *et al.*, 1976; Anglister *et al.*, 1979). Essentially, the enzyme seems to exist in three different molecular forms when freshly prepared extracts of electric organ are analysed by sedimentation centrifugation on sucrose gradients. The different forms sediment at 9, 14·25 and 18·45S for acetylcholinesterase from *Electrophorus* and 7·95, 13·45 and 17·45S for the *Torpedo* enzyme (Rieger *et al.*, 1976). Work on mammalian systems indicates similar molecular forms and the hypothesis has been advanced that the different forms belong to different compartments of the synapse (Gisiger *et al.*, 1978).

Purification of acetylcholinesterase to homogeneity has been achieved using affinity chromatography with quaternary ammonium ligands (e.g. Hopff *et al.*, 1975; Tripathi and O'Brien, 1977). Affinity chromatography purifies a species of acetylcholinesterase with a sedimentation coefficient of 11S. When the different molecular forms are investigated by physicochemical and electron microscopic studies (Anglister *et al.*, 1976; Rieger *et al.*, 1976) the 11S form is found to exist as a tetramer containing four subunits of molecular weight 80 000. The remaining three forms exist as assymetric assemblies of one, two or three tetramers attached to an elongated tail 40–50 nm long. The tail, which is a collagen-like triple helix (Anglister *et al.*, 1979), may serve to anchor the enzyme onto synaptic membranes. The exact structure of the collagenous tail is not clear but it seems to be linked to the catalytic subunits by means of disulphide bonds (Rosenberry and Richardson, 1977).

Acetylcholinesterase seems to be a very antigenic molecule since even trace contamination with this enzyme leads to the production of precipitating titres of antibodies. Thus several antisera raised in Göttingen to membrane fragments derived from the electric organ of *Torpedo*, reacted strongly with acetylcholinesterase, although not more than a total of 50 µg of this enzyme could have been injected over the entire immunization schedule. Many antisera have been prepared to the purified enzyme (Rossier *et al.*, 1975; Riegar *et al.*, 1976; Anglister *et al.*, 1979) and antisera raised to the purified antigen usually give a single immunoprecipitin line on immunodiffusion. Interestingly, one of the earliest antisera to be prepared (Benda *et al.*, 1970) was not monospecific but also contained antibodies to a serum protein. This seems to occur quite often with many antigens due to the highly antigenic nature of serum proteins. Antisera contaminated in this way may easily be purified by adsorption.

In the case of acetylcholinesterase it is easy to identify the immunoprecipitin line corresponding to this enzyme by means of histochemical stains using acetylthiocholine and Fast Red TR to produce a red precipitate (Brogren and Bøg-Hansen, 1975). Eserine may be used at low concentrations to inhibit the formation of product.

When Triton X-100 extracts of *Torpedo* electric organ are analysed with an antiserum to electric organ membrane proteins (Fig. 37) a single rocket

a)
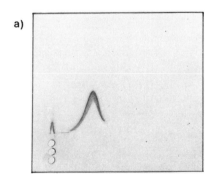

b)
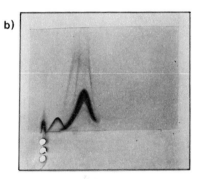

Fig. 37. Immunoelectrophoresis of acetylcholinesterase. A Triton X-100 extract of *Torpedo* electric organ membranes (10 µg protein) was analysed by crossed-rocket immunoelectrophoresis against a polyspecific antiserum raised to *Torpedo* electric organ membrane proteins. In (a) the rocket corresponding to acetylcholinesterase has been stained with a histochemical stain for esterase activity. In (b), the plate has been restained for protein with Coomassie Brilliant Blue. The concentration of antiserum in the gel was 5%, v/v.

is obtained for acetylcholinesterase which suggests that during electrophoresis this enzyme is converted into a homogenous species. A single rocket is also obtained when membrane fragments labelled *in vitro* by reductive methylation are used as antigen. In this case it has been possible to cut out the immunoprecipitin line and analyse it by polyacrylamide gel electrophoresis in the presence of sodium dodecyl sulphate. By means of fluorography the radioactively labelled antigen was found to exist as a single polypeptide of molecular weight 80 000. In this case it seems likely therefore that electrophoresis converts acetylcholinesterase into the 11S form.

Acetylcholinesterase purified from different species possess similar antigenic determinants (Rieger *et al.*, 1976) although it does not seem to be possible to precipitate the enzyme in free solution with heterologous antisera (Fig. 38). Recent work using very sensitive immunological techniques has demonstrated cross-reactivity between the 14S and 18S form of the electric eel enzyme and rat-tail collagen (Anglister *et al.*, 1979). No cross-reactivity was observed with the 11s form of the enzyme and thus it seems clear that the elongated forms of acetylcholinesterase do possess collagenous tails.

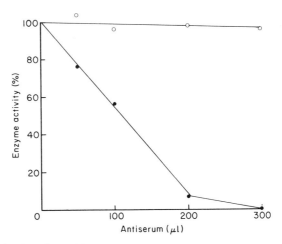

Fig. 38. Immunotitration of acetylcholinesterase activity. An antiserum raised to commercially available *Electrophorus* acetylcholinesterase (Sigma) was used to precipitate the antigen used for the preparation of the antiserum (●) or enzyme present in a Triton X-100 extract of *Torpedo* electric organ (○). The ordinate represents the amount of enzyme activity remaining in the supernatant after storing the antiserum–antigen mixture for 2 days at 4°C and then centrifuging to remove immunoprecipitate.

Immunofluorescence localization of acetylcholinesterase has been performed on cryostat sections of *Electrophorus* electroplax (Benda *et al.*, 1970; Rossier *et al.*, 1975) and also on muscle, brain, and spinal cord (Tsuji *et al.*, 1972). In this way it was shown that the innervated membranes of the electroplax demonstrated much higher fluorescence than the non-innervated side. Certain of the neurones of the spinal cord and brain involved in discharge of the electric organ could also be localized. A well defined histochemical localization procedure for acetylcholinesterase exists but an immunohistochemical approach is preferable in that potentially individual acetylcholinesterase molecules may be localized in the synaptic membranes with ferritin-labelled antibodies, and the immunochemical reagent cannot diffuse away from the enzyme molecule unlike a histo-chemical reaction product.

Many other possible uses exist for antisera to acetylcholinesterase. Studies on the synthesis and degradation of the enzyme may be performed and it may also be possible to use immunoadsorbents to isolate membrane fragments containing the enzyme and thus to obtain an idea of those proteins closely associated with this enzyme. It may also be possible to use this immunochemical approach to remove contaminating membrane frag-ments from other membrane fractions such as synaptic vesicles.

C. Acetylcholine Receptor

Some controversy exists as to the subunit structure of acetylcholine receptor purified from *Torpedo*, one group claiming that this protein contains a single 40 000 molecular weight polypeptide species (Sobel *et al.*, 1977) while others believe in a complex of four subunits of molecular weights 40 000; 50 000; 60 000 and 65 000 (Reed *et al.*, 1975; Witzemann and Raftery, 1978). The most convenient purification procedures for this protein involve affinity chromatography on quaternary ammonium ligands (Olsen *et al.*, 1972; Schmidt and Raftery, 1973) or immobilized snake venom neurotoxins (Karlsson *et al.*, 1972; Olsen *et al.*, 1972; Heilbronn and Mattson, 1974; Salvaterra and Mahler, 1976).

Acetylcholine receptor is very antigenic and immunization of animals with the purified protein leads to a condition very similar to myasthenia-gravis (Heilbronn and Bartfai, 1978), with the injected animals usually developing muscular paralysis soon after a second or third injection of the antigen (Patrick and Lindstrom, 1973). However, immunization with acetylcholine receptor dissociated in SDS is reported to produce antibodies to the receptor without the development of muscular paralysis (Valder-rama *et al.*, 1976). Antisera from animals which develop "experimental autoimmune myasthenia-gravis" seem to be monospecific and to contain sufficient antibodies to enable immunodiffusion and immunoelectrophore-tic studies to be performed (Patrick and Lindstrom, 1973; Sugiyama *et al.*, 1973; Valderrama *et al.*, 1976; Gordon *et al.*, 1977a,b; Teichberg *et al.*, 1977). The immunoprecipitate can be conclusively identified as acetylcho-line receptor since it retains the ability to bind I^{125}-labelled neurotoxin. The bound toxin may then be visualized by means of autoradiography (Teichberg *et al.*, 1977 and Fig. 39).

A wide variety of interesting immunochemical investigations have been performed with antisera to the acetylcholine receptor in attempts to identify the way in which this important protein functions in the process of nerve conduction and also in attempts to understand the neuro-muscular

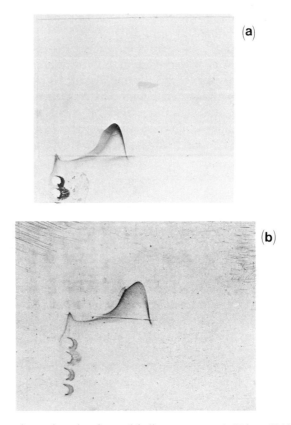

Fig. 39. Immuneolectrophoresis of acetylcholine receptor. A Triton X-100 extract of membranes from *Torpedo marmorata* electric organ (60 μg protein) was analysed by crossed-rocket immunoelectrophoresis against an antiserum raised to acetylcholine receptor purified from *Torpedo californica* by affinity chromatography. Before staining for protein (a) the gel was washed and pressed. The pressed gel was incubated with I^{125}-labelled α-bungarotoxin, rewashed and then dried down. In (b) the autoradiograph of this gel indicates binding of α-bungarotoxin to the major rocket present.

disorder myasthenia-gravis. The many studies on the role of antibodies in this disease are dealt with extensively elsewhere (Heilbronn and Stalberg, 1978; Heilbronn and Bartfai, 1979; Marengo *et al.*, 1979; Niemi *et al.*, 1979).

The phosphorylation of proteins associated with brain membrane fractions has been extensively investigated by Greengard and others (Greengard *et al.*, 1972; Greengard, 1976) and seems to suggest that changes in the level of phosphorylation of specific proteins regulate ion permeability of the postsynaptic membrane. Clearly acetylcholine receptor is intimately involved in this process and indeed phosphorylation of the acetycholine receptor has been shown to occur *in vitro* with membrane fractions prepared from *Electrophorus* (Teichberg *et al.*, 1977) and *Torpedo* (Gordon *et al.*, 1977a,b). In the case of *Torpedo* the results may indicate phosphorylation predominantly of the 65 000 molecular weight subunit, whereas with the *Electrophorus* receptor only a single subunit of molecular weight 49 000 was found to be labelled. For the *Electrophorus* receptor, Teichberg and co-workers first incubated a detergent extract of membrane fragments with P^{32}-labelled ATP and then analysed the resulting mixture by crossed-rocket immunoelectrophoresis with an antiserum to the acetylcholine receptor. A single rocket was obtained and was found to be radioactively labelled by means of autoradiography. When the immunoprecipitate was analysed by polyacrylamide gel electrophoresis in the presence of sodium dodecyl sulphate, radioactive label was found specifically in the 49 000 molecular weight component. The 43 000 and 59 000 subunits were not labelled. These experiments are also important in that they support the belief that acetylcholine receptor is a multisubunit complex. For the *Electrophorus* receptor, for example, a single rocket is obtained which binds α-bungarotoxin (to the 43 000 subunit) and can be phosphorylated (in the 49 000 subunit).

Further interesting observations have been made on the degradation of acetylcholine receptor when mammalian neuromuscular junctions in tissue culture (Kao and Drachman, 1977) or *in vivo* (Stanley and Drachman, 1978) are treated with antisera from patients with myasthenia-gravis. Degradation of acetylcholine receptor was determined from the release of I^{125} from bound I^{125}-labelled α-bungarotoxin and the results clearly demonstrate an increased rate of degradation of the receptor in the presence of myasthenic antibodies. Divalent antibodies are required to produce this enhanced degradation rate. These results perhaps reflect upon the mechanism by which abnormal surface proteins are recognized and destroyed. Thus the binding of IgG interferes with the normal function of the acetylcholine receptor by causing the "capping" of these molecules. This is in some way "sensed" by the cell and thus leads to internalization and destruction of the receptor-antibody complex. Such internalization may occur after actin filaments become associated with the acetycholine receptor in a way similar to that described for lymphocytes and fibroblasts (Singer *et al.*, 1978). Immunohistochemical studies with antisera to acetylcholine receptor and to actin may enable this process of internalization to be studied in greater detail.

Antisera to *Torpedo* and *Electrophorus* acetylcholine receptor have been used to localize this protein in whole electroplax and also in membrane vesicles derived from the electroplax (Karlin *et al.*, 1978). Peroxidase labelled antibodies were used to demonstrate the localization of the receptor predominantly on the innervated membrane of *Electrophorus* electroplax and ferritin-labelled antibodies were used to label specifically those membrane vesicles containing acetycholine receptor in heterogeneous vesicle preparations derived from the electric organ of *Torpedo californica*.

III. Antigens in the Adrenergic Synapse

As with the cholinergic system it is impossible to specifically isolate noradrenergic synaptic vesicles from the brain and difficult to isolate enzymes associated with the synthesis of the adrenergic transmitters. In certain sympathetic nerves it is possible to find sufficient numbers of noradrenergic vesicles to enable significant purification of these structures. Interestingly, two types of noradrenergic vesicles are seen, for example, in the splenic nerve (De Potter and Chubb, 1977; Lagercrantz, 1976) and the hypothesis has been advanced that the large vesicles represent a storage compartment whilst the small vesicles are more directly involved in the secretion of noradrenalin. This is, however, by no means certain. Equally uncertain is the fate of the noradrenergic vesicle after fusion with the presynaptic membrane (De Potter and Chubb, 1977). To investigate these processes at the molecular level it is necessary to purify individual components associated with the noradrenergic vesicle and to investigate the function of these individual components. The adrenal medulla provides a very good model system for studies on the mechanism of exocytosis (Winkler *et al.*, 1974; Winkler, 1977) and it also provides an enriched source of the individual components associated with noradrenergic nerves. Indeed, most of the immunochemical studies performed on proteins and enzymes associated with adrenergic nerves have used antisera raised to antigens purified from the adrenal medulla.

A. *Dopamine β Hydroxylase*

Dopamine β hydroxylase, the enzyme responsible for the synthesis of noradrenalin, is the major protein component of chromaffin granules from the adrenal medulla and has been much studied. It has a subunit molecular weight of 150 000 on polyacrylamide gel electrophoresis in the presence of sodium dodecyl sulphate but without reducing agent. With reducing agent the subunit molecular weight is 75 000. It is very antigenic and, remarkably, monospecific antisera may be obtained by immunizing animals with whole chromaffin granules (Helle *et al.*, 1979). Indeed, the dopamine β hydroxylase molecule is so antigenic that immunization with chromaffin granule membranes gives rise to monospecific antisera against the enzyme, although in this case dopamine β hydroxylase is not the major polypeptide component. This is demonstrated in Fig. 40 where an antiserum to

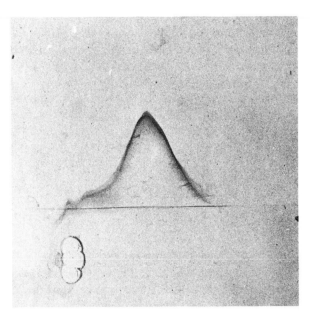

Fig. 40. Crossed immunoelectrophoresis of dopamine β hydroxylase. A Triton X-100 extract of chromaffin granule membranes (10 µg protein) was analysed by crossed-rocket immunoelectrophoresis against an antiserum (4%, v/v) raised to whole chromaffin granule membranes.

chromaffin granule membranes gives a single rocket when analysed against a Triton X-100 extract of chromaffin granule membranes. When chromaffin granule membranes are labelled with [14C]-formaldehyde by reductive methylation an identical rocket is obtained. This rocket contains the subunit associated with dopamine β hydroxylase, as shown when the immunoprecipitate is analysed by polyacrylamide gel electrophoresis in the presence of sodium dodecyl sulphate. The antiserum also inhibits dopamine β hydroxylase activity when tested by means of immunotitration. Commercial availability of the purified enzyme makes immunochemical studies on this enzyme relatively easy, especially since cross-reactivity is obtained between the enzyme from ox adrenal gland and the adrenal glands and brains of other mammalian species (Winkler, 1976; Ross *et al.*, 1978).

Dopamine β hydroxylase has been localized by means of

immunofluorescence in adrenal medulla (Winkler *et al.*, 1974) and in noradrenergic neurones of rat brain (Winkler *et al.*, 1974; Grzanna *et al.*, 1977). Furthermore, axoplasmic flow of this antigen has been demonstrated by immunofluorescence (Nagatsu and Kondo, 1975).

A study on the rate of synthesis of dopamine β hydroxlyase in rat brain has been performed (Ross *et al.*, 1978) with an antiserum to the bovine antigen being used to immunoprecipitate rat brain dopamine β hydroxylase. The authors found that it was necessary to analyse the immunoprecipitates by polyacrylamide gel electrophoresis in the presence of sodium dodecyl sulphate to distinguish between coprecipitants and dopamine β hydroxylase since only 10–15% of the immunoprecipitated radioactivity was in fact dopamine β hydroxylase. They were then able to demonstrate that the two-fold increase in dopamine β hydroxylase activity in noradrenergic cell bodies of the nucleus locus coerulus after administration of reserpine was due to an increase in enzyme amount and not simply a result of enzyme activation.

Antisera to dopamine β hydroxlase have also been used for interesting physiological studies. Thus degeneration of noradrenergic nerve terminals has been found to occur when antibodies to dopamine β hydroxylase are injected into guinea pig tissues (Costa *et al.*, 1976; Rush *et al.*, 1976) and immune lesions can be produced in noradrenergic nerve tracts of rat brain (Blessing *et al.*, 1977) by injecting anti-dopamine β hydroxylase and complement into the third ventricle. Similarly immune lesions are produced in the sympathetic nerves of the rat iris (Costa *et al.*, 1978) by injecting antibodies into the anterior chamber of the eye. The degeneration is mediated by complement since injection of $F_{(ab)_2}$ does not result in degeneration.

Injection of an antiserum to dopamine β hydroxylase into the rat eye has also been used to study retrograde axonal flow of this enzyme (Fillenz *et al.*, 1976). In this case the antiserum was labelled by iodination with I^{125} and movement of antibodies from the iris to the superior cervical ganglion was monitored. This method shows great potential for observing retrograde and normal axoplasmic flow and in particular for the subcellular localization of an antigen during various stages of its "life-cycle".

B. Chromomembrin B

Chromomembrin B is one of the major membrane proteins of the chromaffin granule and has no known enzymatic function. The protein has a molecular weight of 27–28 000 and has been purified from ox chromaffin granule membranes by means of Sephadex chromatography in the presence of sodium dodecyl sulphate (Hörtnagl *et al.*, 1973). Antisera were raised in rabbits immunized with a total of 2·1 mg of the purified protein for each rabbit. The authors could not detect antibodies by means of immunodiffusion procedures and found it necessary to use microcomplement fixation to demonstrate the presence of antibodies against chromomembrin B. This method was also used to demonstrate the presence of cross-reacting material in ox splenic nerve and in adrenal medulla from several other mammalian species. The antisera were also used for the immunohistochemical localization of chromomembrin B in the adrenal medulla (Winkler *et al.*, 1974) at the ultrastructural level by the peroxidase-labelled antibody technique. It was found that only the membranes of the chromaffin granule were labelled in contrast to the results obtained with an antiserum to chromogranin A for which both the membranes and the contents of the chromaffin granules were labelled.

C. Other Adrenergic Antigens

Several other antigens associated with the adrenergic synapse have been listed in Table 7 together with the relevant references. In general the work involves the purification of an antigen, production of a monospecific antiserum and the use of the antiserum for immunocytochemical localization of the antigen.

IV. Summary

The work reviewed briefly in this chapter illustrates the general approach to immunochemical studies on antigens in the nervous system. In cases where a specific protein is chosen for investigation the experimental protocol involves purification of the antigen, production and characterization of an antiserum and then the use of that antiserum. It is hoped that the work discussed in this chapter will help to suggest uses for antisera to other antigens in different parts of the nervous system.

7

Technical Supplement

This chapter aims to provide a concise collection of specific examples, instructions and practical advice based on the material presented elsewhere in this book. The topics described illustrate current immunochemical problems and generally follow the same order as those in the text.

I. Antigen Preparation

A method is described below which may be used to obtain monospecific antisera to protein-subunits starting with relatively crude starting material (Blomberg *et al.*, 1977; Chua and Blomberg, 1979). The method includes:

(1) Partially purifying the antigen of interest or at least preparing a specific subcellular fraction.

(2) Using polyacrylamide gel electrophoresis (with or without sodium dodecyl sulphate, or with cholate or urea depending on the subcellular fraction being examined); or isoelectric focusing in polyacrylamide gels (in the presence or absence of urea) to give optimal purification of the subunit of the antigen of interest.

(3) Staining the gel for protein. Then drying the gel down, cutting out the band of interest and electrophoretically eluting the stained protein, e.g. with the ISCO electrophoretic sample concentrator (Allington *et al.*, 1978) after rehydration of the gel in electrophoresis buffer containing 0·1% (v/v) sodium dodecyl sulphate. With this apparatus the sample is eluted and concentrated.

(4) Removing the Coomassie stain from the protein sample by treating with 0·1 N HCl in 90% acetone at 0°C. In this way 50–100 µg has been prepared for each of several injections.

II. Immunization Details

A. Antigen Amount and Immunization Sites

To prepare a monospecific antiserum in a rabbit, the animal should be immunized with a total of 0·2–1·0 mg of the antigen injected on four or five occasions. On each occasion the antigen should be injected at two or more sites (Fig. 41). Intradermal, subscapular injection sites may be advantageous. To prepare a polyspecific antiserum a total of 1–10 mg of antigen should be used for the immunization schedule.

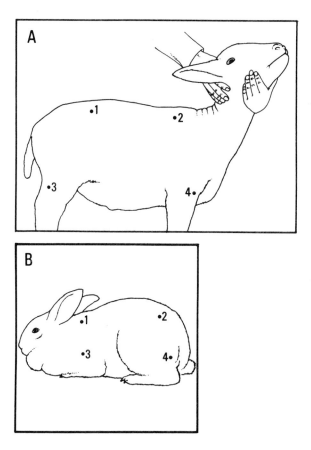

Fig. 41. Recommended sites of injections for multisite injections. A. Sheep or goat. B. Rabbit. Injections are given subcutaneously (1, 2) and intramuscularly (3, 4) and repeated contralaterally, i.e. eight injections in all.

Similar amounts of antigens can be used in both sheep and rabbits although the variation in the immune response to different antigens is so great that no hard and fast rules can be given with respect to the amount of antigen required to produce an antiserum. Indeed in some cases it may be necessary to enhance the immunogenicity of the antigen if an antiserum is to be obtained (see Chapter 2).

One example of an immunization schedule in a sheep is as follows: eight injections of 0·5 ml of antigen preparation emulsified with 0·5 ml of complete Freud's adjuvant at four intramuscular and four subcutaneous sites (Fig. 41A), on four occasions, at two-week intervals, gave excellent precipitating titres to 6-phosphogluconate dehydrogenase, acetyl-CoA carboxylase and fatty acid synthetase (Walker *et al.*, 1976). Blood samples can be processed and the immune response estimated conveniently by immunoprecipitation analyses. Schedules over 8–12 weeks with antigen injection at two-week intervals can give good precipitating titres. It should be pointed out that high precipitating titres are not always required, e.g. for the preparation of immunoadsorbents of low affinity. In this case large blood samples could be obtained regularly (e.g. every two weeks) during an immunization schedule. Blood samples which are collected after shorter immunization schedules often contain far fewer antibodies to contaminating antigens in the antigen preparation of interest.

B. Preparation of Antigen–Adjuvant Mixtures

Exactly equal volumes of adjuvant and antigen solution should be mixed vigorously together until a stable emulsion develops (one which will persist as a drop when placed into water). The most convenient mixing device is a double Luer-lock fitting which enables two syringes to be connected. Very effective mixing of adjuvant and antigen solution can thus be obtained without any loss of material.

III. Bleeding Procedures

Bleeding rabbits from the marginal ear vein is very effective and 5–10 ml of blood may be obtained easily. The rabbit should be wrapped up tightly in a blanket (approx. 150×100 cm) such that only the head and ears are free. While one person holds the animal a second should shave the margin of the upper side of the ear with a scalpel blade and then apply a thin layer of petroleum jelly. The vein may then be sectioned carefully with the scalpel blade or preferably punctured with a needle. After one or two minutes blood will start to flow through the vein and gentle pressure on the vein between the section and the animal's head should ensure that blood will flow from the vein. If the blood flow shows signs of stopping the site of incision may be rubbed with cotton wool which should start the flow of blood again. If difficulties are experienced in obtaining blood then the application of an irritant (e.g. xylene) to the ear in a position distal to the incision will usually induce rapid blood flow. (If xylene is used in this way it should be washed off afterwards with ethanol.) When sufficient blood has been obtained the blood flow may be stopped by gently holding a piece of cotton wool over the wound. In cases where the blood flow is reluctant to stop the cotton wool may be held in place with a paper clip. Blood can rapidly be obtained from sheep or goats by venepuncture of the jugular vein with a syringe needle. This method is useful to obtain a blood volume (10 ml) which is enough for antiserum testing.

Preparative bleeding of rabbits is performed as described above and approx. 40 ml of blood can easily be removed by bleeding from the ear or from the heart. If the animal must be sacrificed most of its blood can be obtained by bleeding from the heart using a cannula connected to a light vacuum.

Preparative bleeding of goats or sheep is easily performed by the Seldinger Wire technique (Fig. 42). A jugular vein is pierced under local anaesthesia (e.g. with 0.5 ml of 2% (v/v)-lignocaine given subcutaneously). After venepuncture with a 14-gauge needle a guide wire is inserted through the needle which allows the subsequent rapid insertion of a catheter over the wire into the jugular vein. A hypodermic syringe (50 ml) may be used to take up to 1 litre of blood which should subsequently be replaced with an equal volume of iso-osmotic saline.

Animals may be rebled at intervals if required. The choice of intervals varies but at least 2–3 weeks should be left between successive bleedings.

IV. Antiserum Processing

Blood is obtained from immunized animals as described above. It is allowed to clot overnight at room temperature and the serum is carefully decanted from the clot. Ammonium sulphate (Fig. 43) is added to the serum at 0°C to give a final concentration of 291 g l^{-1} (50% of saturation). The suspension is centrifuged at 10 000 g for 10 min and the immunoglobulin precipitate is washed at 0°C with a solution of 1·75 M ammonium sulphate until it is white. This procedure will remove albumin, transferrin, and α-proteins including haptoglobin and haemoglobin (Harboe and Ingild, 1973). The final white pellet is dissolved in 10 mM NaH_2PO_4, pH 7·0 and dialysed overnight against water. The precipitated lipoproteins

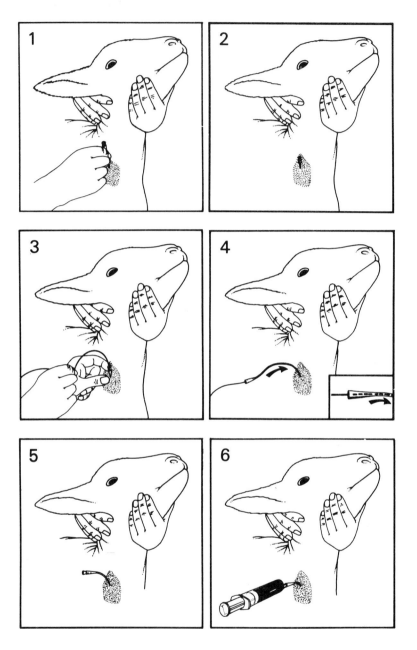

Fig. 42. Bleeding sheep (or goats) from the jugular vein. 1. Piercing of jugular vein with a 14-gauge needle. 2. 14-gauge needle in position. 3. Insertion of guide wire. 4. Insertion of catheter. 5. Catheter (stoppered) in position. 6. Withdrawal of blood (into a 50 ml syringe).

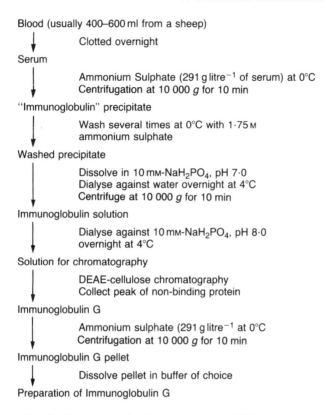

Blood (usually 400–600 ml from a sheep)

Clotted overnight

Serum

Ammonium Sulphate (291 g litre^{-1} of serum) at 0°C
Centrifugation at 10 000 g for 10 min

"Immunoglobulin" precipitate

Wash several times at 0°C with 1·75 M
ammonium sulphate

Washed precipitate

Dissolve in 10 mM-NaH$_2$PO$_4$, pH 7·0
Dialyse against water overnight at 4°C
Centrifuge at 10 000 g for 10 min

Immunoglobulin solution

Dialyse against 10 mM-NaH$_2$PO$_4$, pH 8·0
overnight at 4°C

Solution for chromatography

DEAE-cellulose chromatography
Collect peak of non-binding protein

Immunoglobulin G

Ammonium sulphate (291 g litre^{-1} at 0°C
Centrifugation at 10 000 g for 10 min

Immunoglobulin G pellet

Dissolve pellet in buffer of choice

Preparation of Immunoglobulin G

Fig. 43. Flow diagram for the preparation of IgG from serum.

may be removed by centrifugation at 10 000 g for 10 min. The supernatant is dialysed overnight against 10 mM NaH$_2$PO$_4$ buffer, pH 8·0 and then loaded onto a column (e.g. 4 ml of DEAE-cellulose per ml of serum; Harboe and Ingild, 1973) of DEAE-cellulose previously equilibrated in the same buffer. The column is washed with two column volumes of the buffer and the eluted IgG is concentrated by ammonium sulphate fractionation as described above. Finally, the IgG can be dissolved and dialysed in a buffer of choice for immunochemical work (e.g. 20 mM NaH$_2$PO$_4$, pH 7·0 containing 0·15 M NaCl).

It is advisable to check the proportion of IgG which is eluted from the DEAE-cellulose column by this procedure since it may vary with sera from different species. A suitable way to do this is to elute the column with a linear gradient (10–50 mM) of NaH$_2$PO$_4$ buffer, pH 8·0. This procedure should elute all the immunoglobulins of interest and the fractions containing each immunoglobulin class can be identified by the appropriate commercially available anti-immunoglobulin serum. Non-immune (control) serum should be similarly fractionated for use in comparative experiments with the IgG to the antigen of interest.

V. Preparation of IgG Fragments

The monovalent F_{ab} fragment of IgG is recommended for the localization of intracellular antigens by immunohistochemical techniques (Poole, 1973). The F_{ab} fragment is prepared as follows. First IgG (25 mg ml^{-1}, final concentration) is digested with pepsin (0·5 mg ml^{-1}, final concentration) for 24 h at 40°C in 0·2 M sodium acetate buffer, pH 4·5 containing 0·1% (w/v) sodium azide. Then the pH is adjusted to 8·6 with sodium hydroxide to inactivate the pepsin. After centrifugation the pepsin digest is subjected to chromatography on Sephadex G–200 equilibrated in phosphate-buffered saline. Three peaks should be obtained: first a small IgG peak; second $(F_{ab})_2$ and third F_c. $(F_{ab})_2$ may then be reduced to F_{ab} with 10 mM cysteine for 30 min.

VI. Labelling of IgG and IgG Fragments

For many studies involving the use of antisera it is necessary to use labelled antibody molecules. Antibodies may be labelled by covalently coupling them to other proteins, by making them fluorescent or by labelling them with radioactive reagents.

A. Labelling with other Proteins

In Table 9 four examples are given of proteins which may be covalently attached to IgG or IgG fragments to enable enzyme immune assay or immunohistochemistry to be performed.

B. Fluorescent Antibody

Conjugation with:
    (a) Fluorescein isothiocyanate (Poole, 1973; The and Feltkamp, 1970). To 5 ml of IgG solution (20 mg ml^{-1} in 0·15 M sodium phosphate buffer, pH 9·5) is added 1 mg of fluorescein isothiocyanate isomer 1. After 1 h the reaction products are separated by means of a small Sephadex G–25 column.
    (b) Fluorescamine (Roche, Sigma). To 5 ml of IgG solution (1 mg

Table 9
Labelling IgG and F_{ab} with other proteins

Protein	Method of Linkage	Use	Reference
Alkaline Phosphatase (AP)	5 mg of AP + 2 mg of IgG in 2 ml of phosphate-buffered saline, 0·06% (v/v) glutaraldehyde for 4 h at room temp. Then dialyse against appropriate buffer before use.	enzyme immune assay	Engvall and Perlmann (1971, 1972)
Horse Radish Peroxidase (HRP)	12 mg of HRP + 5 mg of IgG in 1 ml of 0·1 M sodium phosphate, pH 6·8. Add 50 μ of 1% (w/v) glutaraldehyde. Incubate for several hours and then dialyse against appropriate buffer before use.	immuno-histo-chemistry	Avrameas (1969) Kraehenbuhl et al. (1971)
Cytochrome c	8 mg of cytochrome c +5 mg of F_{ab} in 1 ml of 0·1 M sodium phosphate, pH 6·8. Add 50 μl of 1% glutaraldehyde. Incubate for several hours and then dialyse against appropriate buffer before use.	immuno-histo-chemistry	Kraehenbuhl et al. (1971)
Ferritin	For extensive details see Chapter 4.	immuno-histo-chemistry	—

ml^{-1} in 0·2 M sodium borate buffer, pH 9·25) is added 0·05–0·2 ml of fluorescamine (1·5 mg ml^{-1} in acetone) with vortex mixing to ensure immediate mixing. No separation of reaction products is required.

C. Radiolabelled Antibody (and Antigen)

Labelling can be conveniently carried out by:
(a) Reductive methylation (Rice and Means, 1971). To 0·1 mg of

protein in 0·1 ml of 0·2 M sodium borate buffer, pH 9·0 is added 10 μl of 40 mM formaldehyde. Then after 30 s four 2 ml aliquots of sodium borohydride (5 mg ml^{-1}) are added followed after 1 min by a further 10 μl aliquot of sodium borohydride. Either the formaldehyde (^{14}C) or the sodium borohydride (^{3}H) may be radioactive reagents.

(b) Iodination (Landon et al., 1967). To 2 mg of protein in 0·5 ml of phosphate buffered saline in a glass tube add the following: 500 μCi of Na^{125}I, 30 μl of Chloramine T (1 mg ml^{-1}) and mix. After 2 min at room temperature add 30 μl of sodium metabisulphate (2 mg ml^{-1}). Separate the reaction products by gel filtration on Sephadex G–25 or by extensive dialysis.

VII. Immunoprecipitation in Agarose Gels

A. Apparatus

1. *Immunodiffusion.* Immunodiffusion is often performed in agar gels cast in Petri dishes but it is more convenient to use glass plates (10 cm × 10 cm). Smaller plates may be used, e.g. microscope slides. To prevent the gels from drying out they must be kept in a moist environment. Plastic lunch boxes are convenient for this purpose. The immunodiffusion plates are layed on moistened paper tissue or foam rubber in the base of the box. Microscope slides may be placed on a wet paper tissue in a Petri dish.

2. *Immunoelectrophoresis.* Most standard apparatus designed for horizontal electrophoresis may be converted for immunoelectrophoresis (e.g. the Shandon Model U77). Alternatively electrode chambers may be constructed from perspex (approx. dimensions 25 cm × 10 cm × 6 cm) and fitted with platinum electrodes. A cooling plate is required to cool the gel during electrophoresis. Cooling plates may be obtained commercially or constructed from perspex or from copper tubing fixed to a sheet of copper (e.g. 10 cm × 20 cm). Clearly with copper cooling plates electrical insulation is essential: thus the cooling plate may be placed in a plastic bag. A slow steady flow of water through the cooling plate should ensure adequate cooling. Alternatively electrophoresis may be performed in a cold room.

3. *Choice of power pack.* The Shandon SAE 2761 which can be operated on constant voltage up to 400 V is convenient and reliable. The Behring E42/1 which has a similar output but can supply four sets of apparatus simultaneously can also be used. The voltage in the agarose gel can be measured by means of a built in voltmeter and probe with this apparatus.

(iv) A horizontal surface is essential for casting gels. A perspex table may be purchased or constructed which can be adjusted to provide a horizontal surface. In some techniques it is necessary to remove strips of gel after cutting through the agar or agarose gel. A perspex bridge is an advantage here to ensure that a straight line is cut through the gel (see below: "Crossed immunoelectrophoresis"). Well punches may be constructed from stainless steel or rigid plastic tubing of different diameters and connected to a water suction pump. Whatman 3 MM paper is required for electrophoresis wicks and also for pressing gels (see below). Absorbent paper is also required for pressing gels (e.g. Kleenex dressing towel). Plastic trays (approx, $21 \times 11 \times 2$ cm) are required for washing, staining and destaining gels. A boiling-water bath and a water bath set at 50°C are also required. Due to the growing popularity of immunochemical techniques almost all of the apparatus required is commercially available, e.g. from Behring, Pharmacia, LKB and Shandon.

B. Solutions Required

(i) 2% (w/v) Agarose in water (100 ml).

(ii) Immunodiffusion buffer (2 times concentrated).
0·3 M NaCl containing 40 mM-sodium phosphate, pH 7·0; or 0·28 M NaCl containing 103 mM-Tris-HCl, pH 7·6; or 0·16 M-barbitone buffer, pH 8·2. The optimal conditions for immunoprecipitation vary between antibody-antigen systems but it is usual to include 0·15 M NaCl in a gel buffered between pH 6 and 8. For membrane proteins include Triton X–100, Lubrol PX or a similar detergent in the buffers (0·2–1·0%, v/v). Also include sodium azide (0·2%, w/v) to prevent bacterial growth.

(iii) Immunoelectrophoresis buffers

    (a) Running buffers (5 times concentrated)

    "*Svendsen*" *buffer* (Axelsen *et al.*, 1973). Buffer 1: barbitone Na 13 g + barbitol 2·07 g. Boil the water and then add the solids. Make up to 1 litre. Buffer 2: Tris 45·2 g + glycine 56·2 g. Make up to 1 litre. Then mix buffers 1 and 2 to provide a 5-times concentrated stock solution from which the diluted buffer may be made when required.

    Chua and Blomberg (1979) buffer. 5 times concentrated: Tris 48·4 g + sodium acetate 27·22 g + EDTA sodium salt 1·86 g made up to 1 litre after bringing the pH to 8·6 with glacial acetic acid.

    (b) Gel buffers (2 times concentrated)

From the running buffer stock solution take 100 ml and add 150 ml of water plus detergent (e.g. Triton X–100; 0·2%, v/v, final concentration). The presence of non-ionic detergent in the gel is essential for membrane proteins, has no effect upon the resolution of soluble proteins and may be advantageous in later processing of the gel to remove unreacted material.

(iv) Other solutions

0·15 M NaCl to wash out untreated material.

Stain (2 litres)—5 g Coomassie Brilliant Blue (Sigma) + 900 ml of methanol + 200 ml acetic acid + 900 ml water.

Destain (2 litres)—200 ml acetic acid + 900ml methanol + 900 ml water.

Casting Agarose Gels

(E.g. for a 10 × 10 cm glass plate with a gel 1·5 mm thick. Place the bottle containing 2% (w/v) agarose gel into a boiling water bath. Meanwhile pipette a 7·5 ml aliquot of the (×2) gel buffer into a boiling tube and place this in a water bath at 50°C. When the agarose is completely molten transfer 7·5 ml to the boiling tube and mix the two solutions completely. The glass plate must now be "precoated", i.e. dry a thin layer of agarose onto the plate to fix the gel firmly to the glass. Fill about 1/3 of the length of a Pasteur pipette with the 2% (w/v) agarose solution and transfer it quickly onto a glass plate. Working as quickly as you can use another glass plate to spread the agar over the surface. The agar starts to set quite rapidly so do not try spreading for too long. Now dry this thin coat of gel onto the glass plate with a hairdryer (or in an oven). Alternatively simply moisten a paper tissue with the hot agarose and swab the surface of the plate with this. The agarose should dry very rapidly. The gel must now be cast. If antiserum is required in the gel (e.g. for rocket immunoelectrophoresis and Mancini immunodiffusion), it may be added to the agarose in the tube in a water bath at 50°C, e.g. for 1%(v/v) antiserum add 0·15 ml of antiserum to the 15 ml of gel and mix with a glass rod. Lay a glass plate on a horizontal area close to the water bath. Quickly remove the boiling tube from the water bath, wipe the outside of the tube and pour the liquid onto the glass plate. The liquid agarose must be poured as a continuous stream into the centre of the glass plate. Start pouring it onto the plate then increase the rate of flow. Use a glass rod to move the agarose solution to all the edges of the plate, and a Pasteur pipette to remove bubbles from the gel surface. Great care must be taken to ensure that the liquid does not flow over the sides of the plate. Leave the plate for 5-10 min for the gel to set completely. Wells may now be cut in the gel ready for immunodiffusion or immunoelectrophoresis.

When gels are cast on microscope slides, a warm pipette may be used to place 3 ml of agarose directly onto the slide.

D. Procedure for Immunodiffusion

After casting an agarose gel on a 10 × 10 cm glass plate, punch wells according to the pattern required (Fig. 44). Addition of 4% (w/v) polyethylene glycol 4000 may enhance immunoprecipitation (Kostner and Holasek, 1972).

With the Mancini technique ring diameters may be measured after diffusion overnight (e.g. 16 h) or after 1–2 days by which time all of the

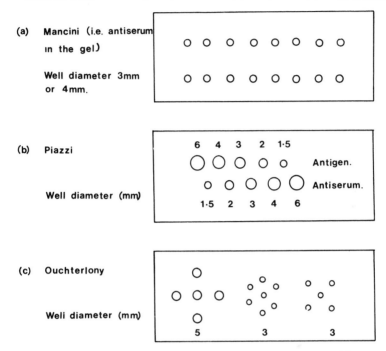

Fig. 44. Well patterns for immunodiffusion. For Mancini immunodiffusion (a) antiserum is incorporated into the agarose gel and antigen diffuses from the well to produce a ring of immunoprecipitate. The diameter of the ring is proportional to the amount of antigen. For Piazzi immunodiffusion (b) well diameters vary such that a very large range of antigen/antibody proportions are tested. In Ouchterlony immunodiffusion (c) one sample of antiserum in the central well may be tested against several antigen samples or *vice versa*.

antigen should have reacted. For the other techniques several days of diffusion may be necessary to visualize all of the antigen–antibody systems present. In all cases it is an advantage to wash and stain the gels for protein as described later.

E. Procedure for Rocket Immunoelectrophoresis

After casting a 10×10 cm plate with agarose gel (agarose is preferred to agar due to its much lower electro-endo-osmosis) containing antiserum, cut out a row of up to 10 wells (4 mm diameter), 0·5 cm apart and 1 cm from the cathode end of the gel. Place the gel onto the cooling plate and attach the Whatman 3 MM wicks (3–5 sheets at each end). The wicks should not overlap onto the wells. With the current switched on (constant voltage, 100 V), place the samples for electrophoresis into the wells. Then place a glass plate on top in such a way as to hold the wicks in contact with the gel,

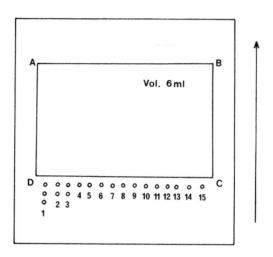

Fig. 45. Rocket immunoelectrophoresis. After casting 15 ml of gel solution onto a 10 × 10 cm glass plate, the section labelled ABCD (5 cm × 8 cm) is removed from the plate and replaced with 6·0 ml of agarose which contains antiserum (i.e. 3 ml of buffer (×2) and 3 ml of agarose (×2)). Wells (2·4 mm; volume 5 µl) are then punched as shown. Electrophoresis is performed overnight at 100 volts (constant voltage at ≤15°C.).

and to prevent evaporation from the gel. Allow electrophoresis to proceed overnight and then process the gel as described below.

An alternative method involves first casting a gel which does not contain antiserum and then removing a section of gel and replacing it with gel containing antiserum (Fig. 45). This method has several advantages: a smaller quantity of antiserum is required; there is no danger of the gel containing antiserum flowing off the plate. The template in Fig. 45 is one pattern that may be used for the analysis of 15 samples. Clearly, if desired, two different antisera could be used in two sections each with a volume of 3·0 ml and each sufficient for the analysis of 7 samples. As illustrated in Fig. 45 larger samples may be applied by increasing the number of wells (e.g. samples 1, 2 and 3) and also by increasing the size of the wells.

Fused rocket immunoelectrophoresis is performed essentially as described for rocket immunoelectrophoresis using the template illustrated in Fig. 46. A second series of wells are included in a staggered array and samples from, for example, a gel filtration column are placed in the wells, allowed to diffuse for 30–60 min and then subject to electrophoresis.

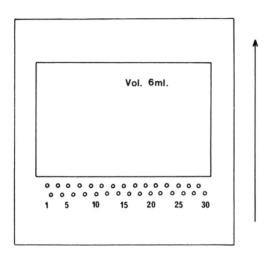

Fig. 46. Fused-rocket immunoelectrophoresis. The procedure for this technique is identical to that adopted for rocket immunoelectrophoresis except that a second row of sample wells are punched. The wells (2·4 mm) are then filled with samples which are allowed to diffuse for 30–60 min prior to electrophoresis overnight (constant voltage, 100 volts at ⩽ 15°C).

F. Procedure for Crossed Immunoelectrophoresis (Weeke, 1973b)

The technique of crossed immunoelectrophoresis involves the electrophoretic separation of a complex protein mixture in a buffered agarose gel, and then another electrophoresis at right angles to the first into a gel containing antibodies which recognize the proteins separated in the first dimension. Thus, for example, an antigen containing preparation may be separated by electrophoresis (Fig. 47a). The area above the dotted line is then covered with gel containing antibodies which recognize the antigen. The filter paper wicks connecting the agarose gel to the electrode chambers are then placed as shown in Fig. 47. Application of a potential difference now results in the proteins being forced into the gel containing antibodies.

The antibodies interact with the antigen to produce an insoluble immuno-precipitate which takes the form of a rocket. The area of the rocket is proportional to the amount of the antigen present. The electrophoresis is

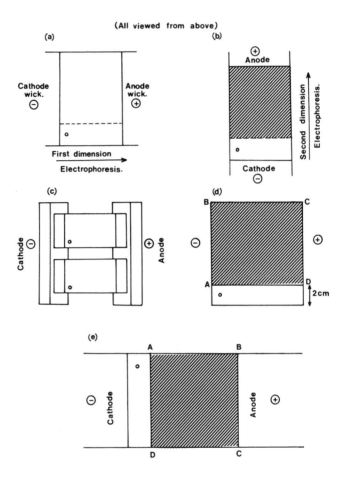

Fig. 47. Crossed-rocket immunoelectrophoresis.

carried out at pH 8·6 since at this pH the antibody molecules have a net zero charge and therefore do not move out of the gel. At this pH most proteins are negatively charged and move towards the anode. For elec-trophoresis in the first dimension, cast a 10 × 10 cm gel without antiserum. Then punch a well in one corner of the gel 1·5 cm from each edge. Now place the gel onto the cooling plate of the electrophoresis apparatus. Take

4–5 (10 × 10 cm) pieces of filter paper and moisten by dipping into the electrode tanks. Use the moistened wicks to connect the gel to the electrode chambers. It is essential that the gel is oriented with the sample well nearest to the cathode chamber. Now place the sample to be analysed into the sample well. Place a glass plate over the wicks in such a way as to

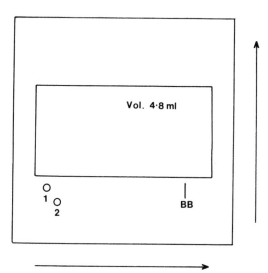

Fig. 48. Crossed-rocket immunoelectrophoresis (alternative method).
Procedure: (i) Cast gel over the whole plate, i.e. 7·5 ml of Agarose (×2) + 7·5 ml of gel buffer (×2).
    (ii) Punch well (1) and analyse the antigen sample by electrophoresis (300 V, constant V) until the bromophenol blue marker dye reaches the point indicated.
    (iii) Cut and remove the section outlined on the template (8 cm × 4 cm) and replace with 4·8 ml of gel solution (2·4 ml of buffer (×2) and 2·4 ml of agarose (×2)) containing serum.
    (iv) Carry out electrophoresis overnight at 100 V, constant voltage into the antiserum-containing gel.
    (v) Well 2 is used for tandem crossed-rocket electrophoresis (i.e. with a second antigen sample) as a means of testing immunochemical identity.
  (BB) Bromophenol blue.

force the wicks into contact with the gel and thus establish good electrical contact. Two plates may be run at the same time if desired (Fig. 47c). When both samples have been applied place the cover over the apparatus and switch on the power pack. Adjust the voltage to 300 V (constant voltage) and leave for 1·5 h. When the first electrophoresis step is completed, switch off the power and remove the plate from the electrophoresis apparatus. Leave the wicks in the apparatus. You must now remove most of the gel from the plate as shown in Fig. 47d. The shaded area must be removed. This is achieved as follows. First cut along line A–D using a perspex bridge to guide the scalpel blade. Then remove the bridge and use the scalpel to lift the gel away from the plate at corner C (or D). Carefully peel the gel from the plate taking care not to disturb the gel below the line A–B. Discard the gel you have removed and put the plate on the horizontal surface. Now go to the water bath and pipette the amount of

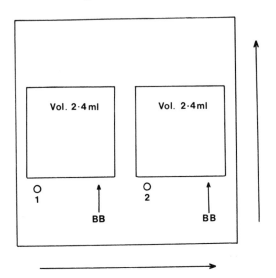

Fig. 49. Crossed-rocket Immunoelectrophoresis (for two samples). The procedure is identical to that described in the previous figure with the exception that two samples are analysed. Electrophoresis in the first dimension is completed in approximately 45 minutes and then two sections of agarose gel (4 cm × 4 cm) containing antiserum (1·2 ml of buffer (×2) and 1·2 ml agarose (×2)) are cast before electrophoresis overnight in the second dimension. (BB) Bromophenol blue.

antiserum required into the 12 ml of melted gel (6 ml of gel buffer (×2) + 6 ml of 2% agarose). Mix well by stirring with a glass rod. Remove the boiling tube from the water bath and quickly take it and pour the agarose onto the glass plate as before. Pour the agarose solution onto the plate in such a way as to prevent gel flowing onto the gel already present. Leave about 10 min for the gel to set. Section ABCD (Fig. 47d) should now be covered with gel containing antibodies. The plate must now be put back into the electrophoresis apparatus oriented as shown in Fig. 47c. Place the wicks in position and the glass plate on top. Then replace the cover over the electrophoresis apparatus and switch the power pack on. Adjust the "voltage" to read 100 V, and leave overnight at ≤15°C.

Alternatively, as with rocket immunoelectrophoresis, it is usually an advantage to use a template (Figs 48 and 49) to produce antiserum-containing gel sections. It is also a good idea to mix biomorphenol blue tracking dye with the sample. The first dimension separation may then be terminated when the dye reaches the point marked (BB) in Figs 48 and 49.

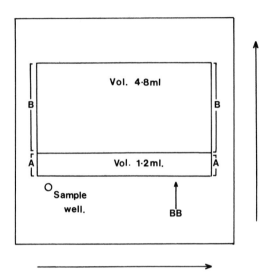

Fig. 50. Crossed immunoelectrophoresis with intermediate gel.
  (i) Cast 15 ml of gel solution without antiserum and analyse the antigen sample by electrophoresis in the first dimension.
 (ii) Remove that section of gel labelled A (1 cm × 8 cm) and replace with buffered agarose containing e.g. pure antigen or mono-specific antiserum (0·6 ml of buffer (×2) and 0·6 ml of agarose (×2)).
(iii) When section A has set, cut around and remove section B (8 cm × 4 cm). Replace this with 4·8 ml of gel containing a second antiserum (2·4 ml of buffer (×2) and 2·4 ml of agarose (×2)).
(BB) Bromophenol blue.

Intermediate gels containing antigen or antiserum may also be used as in Fig. 50. Here, after a first dimension separation by electrophoresis, an intermediate gel is cast between the separated antigen and the antiserum-containing gel. If the intermediate gel contains pure antigen or an antiserum of defined specificity the antigens recognized by the second antiserum (in gel section B) may be identified.

In Fig. 51 a general procedure is outlined which enables a strip of polyacrylamide gel containing separated antigens to be analysed by crossed-rocket immunoelectrophoresis. The antigens may be separated by polyacrylamide gel electrophoresis or by isoelectric focusing (Chua and Blomberg, 1979).

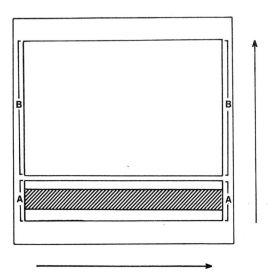

Fig. 51. Crossed immunoelectrophoresis with polyacrylamide gel first dimension.
Procedure: (i) Cast gel over whole plate i.e. 7·5 ml agarose (×2) and 7·5 ml gel buffer (×2).
  (ii) Cut out the two section outlines on the template (A and B).
  (iii) Fill in the upper section (B: 6 cm × 9 cm) with a mixture of 4 ml of agarose (×2), 4 ml of gel buffer (×2), Triton X-100 (1% v/v, final concentration) and polyethylene glycol (4% v/v).
  (iv) Fill in the lower section (A: 1·8 cm × 9 cm) as follows:
    (a) place a strip of polyacrylamide (1 mm thick in the position shown (cross-hatched area).
    (b) cover the strip with 2·0 ml of 1% agarose made by mixing 1·0 ml of agarose (×2) with 1·0 ml of gel buffer (×2) containing 2% (w/v) sodium deoxycholate.
  (v) Perform electrophoresis overnight at 100 V (constant voltage) at ⩽ 15°C.

When the first dimension separation is performed in high ionic strength buffer (e.g. Laemli system) the strip of gel should be incubated for 15–30 min in water before performing the second dimension electrophoresis.

G. Staining Gels for Protein

Immunoprecipitates are often visible as white lines in the gel when viewed against a dark background. However, for increased sensitivity it is usual to stain the gel for protein; some immunoprecipitates are not seen without staining. Another advantage of processing the gel is that it yields a permanent and easily stored record.

After electrophoresis the gel contains a large amount of protein other than that in the immunoprecipitate (e.g. unreacted antibody molecules and non-immune IgG). This protein is removed by pressing and washing the gel. Take the gel and fill the sample well with a drop of saline. Lay the gel on a bench and place a 10 × 10 cm square of Whatman 3 MM paper over it taking care not to trap any air. Place a pad of absorbent paper (approx. 50 × 50 cm) folded four times to give a pad (approx. 10 × 10 cm) over this, then a glass plate and finally a 1 kg weight (reagent bottle etc). Leave for 10 min, then remove the weight, the absorbent paper and the Whatman filter paper. Great care is required in removing the Whatman paper square to prevent the gel being removed from the surface of the glass plate. Now immerse the pressed gel in the saline and leave for 20 min. Then pour off the saline carefully. The gel may float free of the glass plate. Pour more saline into the tray and leave the gel for a further 20 min. Again carefully pour off the saline and replace it with distilled water; leave for 20 min. Carefully remove the plate and gel from the tray and press it as described above. After removing the Whatman paper square, dry the gel onto the glass plate with a hairdryer or in an oven. Place the plate into the empty tray and cover the plate with Coomassie blue stain. Leave for 20 min and then pour the stain away. Rinse the plate in distilled water and then add destaining solution. Agitate and replace destaining until the plate shows blue rockets against a reasonably colourless background. Then pour off the destain and dry the plate.

VIII. Techniques for the Identification of Antigens in Immunoprecipitation Lines

A wide variety of techniques may be used to decide which of several immunoprecipitation lines obtained with a multispecific antiserum corresponds to an antigen of interest. Some useful techniques are illustrated below. They serve to show the novelty and ingenuity which has been used to approach the problem of identifying an immunoprecipitation line to an antigen of interest. Several immunodiffusion and immunoelectrophoretic techniques have been previously described in several places in the book, by which reactions of identity of a purified antigen (or monospecific antiserum) with an unidentified antigen may be carried out. These techniques will not be considered here.

Staining of immunoprecipitation lines has been extensively used to identify antigens. For many enzymes simple histochemical staining methods exist. A list of the more common techniques is shown in Table 10.

Table 10
A selection of enzyme stains

Enzyme type	Reagent	Reference	Notes
Dehydro genase	substrate + NAD(P) + p-Nitro Blue Tetrazolium	Walker et al., (1976)	—
Esterase	naphthyl acetate + Fast Red TR	Brogren and Bøg-Hansen (1975)	e.g. acetyl choline esterase
Nucleotide phosphatase	substrate + Pb(NO$_3$)$_2$ + (NH$_4$)$_2$S	Blomberg and Perlman (1971b)	e.g. AMP, ADP, ATP phosphatases
Oxidase	p-phenylene-diamine	Uriel (1964)	—
phosphatase (acid or alkaline)	α-naphthyl phosphate + Fast Blue B	Blomberg and Perlman (1971a)	—
Peroxidase	(a) benzidine + H$_2$O$_2$ (b) α-naphthol + phenylenediamine (NADI)	Uriel (1964)	— / e.g. cytochrome oxidase

Many other histochemical stains have been used and are described by Owen and Smith (1977). Enzyme activity may be measured in the test tube with cut-out immunoprecipitation lines. If this technique is used it is advisable to carry out immunodiffusion or immunoelectrophoresis in duplicate, so that one plate can be stained for protein and used as a guide for the localization of the otherwise invisible immmunoprecipitation lines. Immunoprecipitation lines can be identified by binding of radiolabelled ligands. Examples of these procedures are shown in Table 11.

Several techniques have been developed by which antigens radiolabelled *in vivo* or *in vitro* can be identified. Antigens which are radiolabelled may be subjected to immunodiffusion or immunoelectrophoresis. The individual immunoprecipitates may be analysed by polyacrylamide gel electrophoresis in the presence of sodium dodecyl sulphate or by isoelectric focusing in 9 M urea. If the subunit molecular weight or isoelectric point of an antigen are known the immunoprecipitate can be identified. This approach may be used in reverse where protein analysis is carried out first and a known protein subunit is then subjected to immunochemical analysis.

Table 11
Identification of antigen of interest by binding of radiolabelled ligands

Ligand	Antigen(s)	Reference
^{125}I-Bungarotoxin	Acetylcholine receptor	Teichberg et al. (1977)
^{14}C-Epinephrine	Plasma membrane proteins	Blomberg and Berzins (1975)
^{32}P-phosphate	casein	Al-Sarraj et al. (1978)
	Acetylcholine receptor	Gordon et al. (1977)
	Acetylcholine receptor	Teichberg et al. (1977)

Table 12
Methods for the preparation of immunoadsorbents

Gel type	Activation with	Reference	Comments
Sepharose	cyanogen bromide	Porath et al. (1973)	the activated gel is commercially available
Sepharose	epichloro-hydrin	Porath and Sundberg (1970)	gives highly cross-linked gel
Aminohexyl ⎫ Sepharose Carboxyhexyl ⎭	carbodimide	Lowe and Dean (1974)	—
Aminoethyl-Biogel P-150	4 simple steps	Fiddler and Gray (1978)	—
Cellulose	azide	Miles and Hales (1968a, b)	—

IX. Preparation of Immunoadsorbents

Antibodies (and antigens) may be immobilized by a wide variety of methods. A selection of methods is presented in Table 12. In addition a

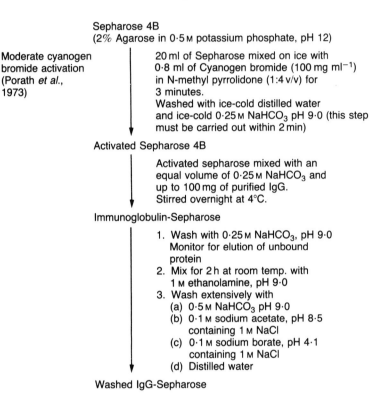

Sepharose 4B
(2% Agarose in 0·5 M potassium phosphate, pH 12)

Moderate cyanogen bromide activation (Porath *et al.*, 1973)

20 ml of Sepharose mixed on ice with 0·8 ml of Cyanogen bromide (100 mg ml⁻¹) in N-methyl pyrrolidone (1:4 v/v) for 3 minutes.
Washed with ice-cold distilled water and ice-cold 0·25 M NaHCO₃ pH 9·0 (this step must be carried out within 2 min)

Activated Sepharose 4B

Activated sepharose mixed with an equal volume of 0·25 M NaHCO₃ and up to 100 mg of purified IgG.
Stirred overnight at 4°C.

Immunoglobulin-Sepharose

1. Wash with 0·25 M NaHCO₃, pH 9·0 Monitor for elution of unbound protein
2. Mix for 2 h at room temp. with 1 M ethanolamine, pH 9·0
3. Wash extensively with
   (a) 0·5 M NaHCO₃ pH 9·0
   (b) 0·1 M sodium acetate, pH 8·5 containing 1 M NaCl
   (c) 0·1 M sodium borate, pH 4·1 containing 1 M NaCl
   (d) Distilled water

Washed IgG-Sepharose

Fig. 52. Preparation of a sepharose immunoadsorbent.

wide variety of other gel types are commercially available from Bio-Rad (e.g. Affigel 10 which is preactivated; Affigels 701 and 702 which have smaller beads than conventional matrices); Pharmacia and LKB.

Usually immunoadsorbents are prepared by reacting proteins with cyanogen bromide-activated Sepharose. The procedure involved is given in detail in Fig. 52.

It is recommended that immunoadsorbents are prepared from antisera obtained early in immunization schedules. In this way antibodies of relatively low affinity are immobilized and thus the antigen can be eluted from the coloumn under less denaturing conditions. A variety of conditions may be used to elute bound antigen: electrophoresis (with or without denaturing agents, e.g. urea and sodium dodecyl sulphate); buffers at low pH (e.g. 0.2 M Glycine-HCl pH 2.8); strong salt solutions (e.g. 5 M magnesium chloride); chaotropic agents (e.g. 3 M lithium isothiocyanate); strongly denaturing agents (e.g. urea and sodium dodecyl sulphate). It is recommended that the antigen is eluted from the immunoadsorbent as soon as possible after application of the sample.

X. Staphylococcal Protein A-antibody adsorbent

The specific and strong interaction of protein A with serum immunoglobulin (Ig) has been known since Jensen (1959) isolated protein A from the cell walls of *Staphylococcus aureus*. Subsequently the reactive ligand was identified as the F_c portion of IgG molecules (Forsgren and Sjöquist, 1966; Kronvall and Frommel, 1970). The proportion of serum globulins which is bound by protein A has been reported to vary from more than 90% in rabbits to a minor proportion of immunoglobulin molecules in sheep and goats (Lind *et al.*, 1970; Kronvall *et al.*, 1970). However, rabbit, sheep, goat and mouse polyspecific antisera to mouse and human immunoglobulins (Ig) were all similarly effective in binding to *Staphylococcus aureus* cells, when used to give immune complexes with Ig in detergent-solubilized mouse or human lymphocytes (Kessler, 1976). This study indicates that the staphylococcal adsorbent performs well with antibody-complexes, involving antisera from mammalian species whose serum immunoglobulins do not react with protein A as quantitatively as do those of rabbits (Kessler, 1976).The binding phenomenon means that protein A or protein A-containing *Staphylococcus aureus* can be used as an anti-immunoglobulin (IgG) reagent. Protein A-containing *Staphylococcus aureus* was initially used in a radioimmunoassay to quantitate $\propto$-faetoprotein in normal adult serum (Jonsson and Kronvall, 1974).

The increasing need for rapid specific immunoisolation methods to isolate soluble and membrane antigens in many fields of cell biology led to detailed studies of the use of Cowan I strain of *Staphylococcus aureus* as an immunoadsorbent for antibodies complexed with radiolabelled antigens from mammalian cell lysates. The studies culminated in the development of a technique where protein A-bearing strains of the bacterium could be substituted for a second antibody in indirect double antibody immune precipitation reactions (Kessler, 1975).

Immune complexes are rapidly (within seconds) tightly bound to the protein A-containing bacteria, whereas maximum binding of free IgG is a much slower process. Tight binding of immune complexes means that bacterial washing procedures may be conveniently carried out before antigen elution. The elution of antigen can be achieved with a number of denaturing reagents. The final analytical step of most immunoisolation procedures is polyacrylamide gel electrophoresis in the presence of SDS. Antigens are therefore eluted from the bacteria by methods giving preparations ready for electrophoresis, e.g. by treatment with sample-volumes of SDS-urea and reducing agent (Kessler, 1976). The bacteria are simply pelleted by low speed centrifugation and the antigen-containing sample is then immediately ready for electrophoresis.

With two provisos this technique is to be generally recommended for soluble or membrane antigen isolation. The first requirement is that antibodies in a specific antiserum should have high affinities for protein

Cells in monolayer culture

    incubate with [^{35}S]-methionine to label proteins for 15 min at 37°C

[^{35}S]-"labelled" cells

    incubate with 10 mM trinitrobenzene sulphonic acid (TNBS) for 30 min at 40°C in phosphate-buffered saline pH 7·8. Wash cells in phosphate-buffered saline, pH 7·8.

TBNS-derivatized [^{35}S]-"labelled" cells

    incubate at 4°C for 20 min in phosphate-bufffed saline, pH 7·8 containing rabbit anti-DNP (dinitrophenyl) IgG (0·5 mg ml) and 1 mg ml^{-1} of bovine serum albumin.

Anti-DNP-Trinitrophenyl (TNP)-[^{35}S]-"labelled" cells

    Cells washed with phosphate-buffered saline, scraped from plate, sedimented, and lysed with phosphate buffered saline (200 µl) containing 0·5% Nonidet P-40 and protease inhibitors.

Cell lysate

    Centrifuge at low speed to obtain plasma membrane protein containing supernatant. Incubate supernatant with 100 µl of 10% (wt/vol) formaldehyde-fixed heat killed *S. aureus* for 15 min at 4°C in 12·5 mM potassium phosphate buffer, pH 7·4 containing 0·2 M NaCl, 0·02% NaN$_3$ and 1 mg ml^{-1} of bovine serum albumin.

S. aureus-Anti-DNP-TNP-[^{35}S]-labelled externally oriented membrane proteins

    1. Wash in sequence with incubation buffer, 0·1% SDS, 0·05% Nonidet P-40 and finally with incubation buffer.
    2. Wash bacteria with electrophoresis sample buffer containing 2% SDS and 40 mM dithiothreitol ± 6 M urea. Sediment bacteria.

TNP-[^{35}S]-labelled externally oriented membrane proteins for polyacrylamide gel electrophoresis

Fig. 53. Immunoisolation of externally oriented membrane antigens with protein A-bearing *Staphylococcus aureus*

A-bearing *Staphylococcus aureus* (e.g. with antisera from sheep and goats).The second requirement is that non-specific adsorption should be minimal. A convenient and novel scheme for the immunoisolation of externally oriented membrane antigens involving the use of *Staphylococcus aureus* is shown in Fig. 53. This scheme has been adapted from the method described by Kaplan *et al*. (1979).

An alternative to protein A-bearing *Staphylococcus aureus* is the use of protein A-Sepharose. Protein A-Sepharose has been prepared and allowed to react with antibodies to a subunit of cytochrome oxidase. After covalent binding of the antibodies to the protein A-Sepharose the immunoadsorbent has been elegantly used to isolate cytochrome oxidase precursors (Werner and Machleidt,1978).

References

Abuchowski, A., Van Es, T., Palczuk, N. C. and Davis, F. F. (1977a). *J. Biol. Chem.* **252**, 3578–3581.

Abuchowski, A., McCoy, J. R., Palczuk, N. C., Van Es, T. and Davis, F. F. (1977b). *J. Biol. Chem.* **252**, 35832–3586.

Adair, W. S., Jurvich, D., and Goodenough, U. W. (1978). *J. Cell. Biol.* **79**, 281–285.

Addison, G. M. and Hales, C. N. (1971). *Horm. Metab. Res.* **3**, 59–60.

Alberts, A. W., Strauss, A. W., Hennessy, S. and Vagelos, P. R. (1975). *Proc. Natl. Acad. Sci. USA* **72**, 3956–3960.

Allington, W. B. Cordry, A. L., McCullough, G. A., Mitchell, D. E. and Nelson, I. W. (1978). *Anal. Biochem.* **85**, 188–196.

Al-Sarraj, K., White, D. A. and Mayer, R. J. (1978). *Biochem. J.* **173**, 877–883.

Al-Sarraj, K., Newbury, J., White, D. A. and Mayer, R. J. (1979). *Biochem J.* **182**.

Anglister, L., Rogozinski, S. and Silman, I. (1976). *FEBS Lett* **69**, 129–132.

Anglister, L., Tarrab-Hazdai, R., Fuchs, S. and Silman, I. (1979). *Eur. J. Biochem.* **94**, 25–29.

Arnon, R. (1971). *In* "Current Topics in Microbiology and Immunology," Vol. 54, pp. 47–93. Springer-Verlag, Berlin.

Arnon, R. (1973). *In* "The Antigens" Vol. 1, (M. Sela, Ed.) pp. 87–159. Academic Press, New York and London.

Avrameas, S. (1969). *Immunochemistry* **6**, 43–52.

Avrameas, S. and Ternynck, T. (1969).

Axelsen, N. H., Bock. E. and Krøll, J. (1973). *In* "A Manual of Quantitative Immunoelectrophoresis, (N. H. Axelsen, J. Krøll and B. Weeke, Eds.), pp. 91–94. Universitetsforlaget, Oslo.

Beeley, J. G. (1976). *Biochem. J.* **155**, 345–351.

Benda, P., Tsuji, S., Daussant, J. and Changeux, J. P. (1970). *Nature* **225**, 1149–1150.

Berzins, K., Lando, P., Raftell, M. and Blomberg, F. (1977a). *Biochim. Biophys. Acta* **497**, 337–348.

Berzins, K., Lando, P., Raftell, M. and Blomberg, F. (1977b). *Biochim. Biophys. Acta* **481**, 586–593.

Betts, S. A. and Mayer, R. J. (1975). *Biochem. J.* **151**, 263–270.

Betts, S. A. and Mayer, R. J. (1977). *Biochim. Biophys. Acta* **496**, 302–311.

Bjerrum, O. J. and Bøg-Hansen, T. C. (1976a). *Biochim. Biophys. Acta* **455,** 66–89.

Bjerrum, O. J. and Bøg-Hansen, T. C. (1976b). *In:* "Biochemical Analysis of Membranes", (A. H. Maddy, Ed.), pp. 378–426, Chapman & Hall, London.

Bjerrum, O. J., Lundahl, P., Brogren, C-H. and Hjerten, S. *Biochim. Biophys. Acta* (1975), **394,** 173–181.

Blessing, W. W., Costa, M., Geffen, L. B., Rush, R. A. and Fink, G. (1977). *Nature* **267,** 368–369.

Blobel, G. (1977) *In:* "Gene Expression" (B. F. C. Clark, H. Klenow and J. Zeuthen, Eds), pp. 99–108. Pergamon Press, Oxford.

Blomberg, F. and Berzins, K. (1975). *Eur. J. Biochem.* **56,** 319–326.

Blomberg, F. and Perlmann, P. (1971a). *Exp. Cell Res.* **66,** 104–112.

Blomberg, F. and Perlman, P. (1971b). *Biochim. Biophys. Acta* **233,** 53–60.

Blomberg, F., Cohen, R. S. and Siekevitz, P. (1977). *J. Cell. Biol.* **74,** 204–255.

Bock, E. (1978). *J. Neurochem.* **30,** 7–14.

Bock, K. W. and Matern, S. (1973). *Eur. J. Biochem.* **38,** 20–24.

Bolton, A. E. and Hunter, W. M. (1973). *Biochim. Biophys. Acta* **329,** 318–330.

Borgese, N. and Meldolesi, J. (1976). *FEBS Letts.* **63,** 231–234.

Bouma, H. and Fuller, G. M. (1975). *J. Biol. Chem.* **250,** 4678–4683.

Brandon, C. and Wu, J.-Y. (1978). *J. Neurochem.* **30,** 791–797.

Brandt, J., Elde, R. P. and Goldstein, M. (1979). *Neuroscience.* **4,** 249–270.

Brogren, C. H. and Bøg-Hansen, T. C. (1975). *Scand. J. Immunology,* **4,** Supplement 2, 35–51.

Brownsey, R. W., Hughes, W. A., Denton, R. M. and Mayer, R. J. (1977). *Biochem. J.* **168,** 441–445.

Burridge, K. (1978). *In* "Methods in Enzymology" Vol. L, (V. Ginsburg, Ed.), pp. 54–64. Academic Press, New York and London.

Cahill, A. L. and Morris, S. J. (1979). *J. Neurochem.* **32,** 855–867.

Cailla, H. L., Vannier, C. J. and Delaage, M. A. (1976). *Anal. Biochem.* **70,** 195–202.

Catt, K. and Tregear, G. W. (1967). *Science* **158,** 1570–1572.

Chan, S. H. P. and Tracy, R. P. (1978). *Eur. J. Biochem.* **89,** 595–606.

Chao, L. P. (1975). *J. Neurochem.* **25,** 261–766.

Chao, L. P., Wolfgram, F J. and Eng, L. F. (1977). *Neurochem. Res.* **2,** 323–325

Cho-Chung, Y. S. and Pitot, H. C. (1968). *Eur. J. Biochem.* **3,** 401–406.

Chua, N. H. and Blomberg, F. (1979). *J. Biol. Chem.* **254,** 215–233.

Cinader, B. (1963). Immunochemistry of enzymes. *Ann. N.Y. Acad. Sci.* **103,** 495–548.

Cinader, B. (1967). *In* "Antibodies to Biologically Active Molecules", (B. Cinader, Ed.) pp. 85–137, Pergamon, Oxford.

Cinader, B. (1977). *In* "Methods in Immunology and Immunochemistry", Vol. IV (C. A. Williams and M. W. Chase, Eds), pp. 313–375. Academic Press, New York and London.

Cinader, B. and Lafferty, K. J. (1964). *Immunol.* **7,** 342–362.

Clausen, J. (1971). *In* "Laboratory Techniques in Biochemistry and Molecular Biology", pp. 443–444. North Holland, Amsterdam.

Collins, W. P. and Hennam, J. F. (1976). *In* "Molecular Aspects of Medicine", Vol. 1, H. Baum and J. Gergely, Eds), pp. 3–128. Pergamon, Oxford.

Converse, C. A. and Papermaster, D. S. (1975). *Science* **189,** 469–472.

Costa, M., Furness, J. B., Geffen, L. B., Lewis, S. Y. and Rush, R. A. (1978). *J. Anat.* **126**, 652.

Costa, M., Rush, R. A., Furness, J. B. and Geffen, L. B. (1976). *Neurosci. Lett.* **3**, 201–207.

Creighton, W. D., Lambert, P. H. and Miescher, P. A. (1973). *J. Immunol.* **111**, 1219–1227.

Crumpton, M. J. and Parkhouse, R. M. E. (1972). *FEBS Lett.* **22**, 210–212.

Dale, G. and Latner, A. L. (1969). *Clin. Chim. Acta* **24**, 61.

Dean, P. D. G., Brown, P., Leyland, M. J., Watson, D. H., Angal, S. and Harvey, M. J. (1977). *Biochem. Soc. Trans.* 1111–1113.

Dennick, R. G. and Mayer, R. J. (1977). *Biochem. J.* **161**, 167–174.

De Potter, W. P. and Chubb, I. W. (1977). *Neuroscience* **2**, 167–174.

Don, M. and Masters, C. J. (1975). *Biochem. Biophys. Acta* **384**, 25–36.

Edelman, G. M. and Rutishauser, U. (1974). *In* "Methods in Enzymology", Vol. 34, (W. B. Jakoby and M. Wilchek, Eds.) pp. 195–225, Academic Press, New York and London.

Ekwall, K., Söderholm, J. and Wadström, T. (1976). *J. Immunol. Methods,* **12**, 103–115.

Eng, L. F., Uyeda, C. T., Chao, L. P. and Wolfgram, F. (1974). *Nature* **250**, 243–245.

Engall, E. and Perlmann, P. (1971). *Immunochemistry* **8**, 871–874.

Engall, E. and Perlmann, P. (1972). *J. Immunol.* **109**, 129–135.

Fiddler, M. B. and Gray, G. R. (1978). *Anal. Biochem.* **86**, 716–724.

Fillenz, M., Gagnon, C., Stoeckel, K. and Thoenen, H. (1976). *Brain Res.* **114**, 293–303.

Forsgren, A. and Sjöquist, J. (1966). *J. Immunol.* **97**, 822–827.

Fuxe, K., Hökfelt, T., Eneroth, P., Gustafsson, J.-A. and Skett, P. (1977). *Science* **196**, 899–900.

Galfre, G., Howe, S. C., Milstein, C., Butcher, G. W. and Howard, J. C. (1977). *Nature* **266**, 550–552.

Ghangas, G. S. and Milman, G. (1977). *Science* **196**, 1119–1120.

Gilbert, D. (1978). *Nature* **272**, 577–578.

Gintzler, A. R., Gersham, M. D. and Spector, S. (1978). *Science* **199**, 447–448.

Gisiger, V., Vigny, M., Gautron, J. and Rieger, F. (1978). *J. Neurochem.* **30**, 501–516.

Gordon, A. S., Davis, C. G. and Diamond, I. (1977a). *Proc. Natl. Acad. Sci.* **74**, 263–267.

Gordon, A. S., Davis, C. G., Milfay, D. and Diamond, I. (1977b). *Nature* **267**, 539–540.

Grabar, P. and Williams, C. A. (1953). *Biochim. Biophys. Acta* **10**, 193–194.

Greengard, P. (1976). *Nature* **260**, 101–108.

Greengard, P., McAfee, D. A. and Kebabian, J. W. (1972) *In* "Advances in Cyclic Nucleotide Research". Vol. I (P. Greengard, R. Paoletti and G. A. Robinson, Eds), pp. 337–355. Raven Press, New York.

Griesser, G. H. (1978). *Neuroscience* **3**, 301–306.

Grzanna, R., Morrison, J. H., Coyle, J. T. and Molliver, M. E. (1977). *Neurosci. Lett.* **4**, 127–134.

Haase, W., Schäfer, A., Murer, H. and Kinne, R. (1978). *Biochem. J.* **172**, 57–62.

Hackenbrock, C. R. and Hammon, K. M. (1975). *J. Biol.* **250**, 9185–9197.

Hamaguchi, Y., Kato, K., Fukui, H., Shirakawa, I., Okawa, S., Ishikawa, E., Kobayashi, K. and Katunuma, N. (1976a). *Eur. J. Biochem.* **71**, 459–467.

Hamaguchi, Y., Kato, K., Ishikawa, E., Kobayashi, K. and Katunuma, N. (1976b). *FEBS Lett.* **69**, 11–14.

Harboe, N. and Ingild, A. (1973). *In* "A Manual of Quantitative Immunoelectrophoresis", N. H. Axelsen, J. Krøll and B. Weeke, Eds), pp. 161–164, Universitetsforlaget, Oslo.

Hardwicke, P. M. D. (1976). *Biochim. Biophys. Acta* **422**, 357–364.

Hartman, B. C., Zide, D. and Udenfriend, S. (1972). *Proc. Nat. Acad. Sci.* **69**, 2722–2726.

Haustein, D. and Warr, G. W. (1976). *J. Immunol. Meth.* **12**, 323–336.

Heidelberger, M. and Kendall, F. E. (1929). *J. Exp. Med.* **50**, 809–823.

Heidmann, T. and Changeaux, J. P. (1978). *Annu. Rev. Biochem.* **47**, 317–357.

Heilbronn, E. and Bartfai, T. (1978). *Prog. Neurob.* **11**, 171–188.

Heilbronn, E. and Mattson, C. (1974). *J. Neurochem.* **22**, 315–317.

Heilbronn, E. and Stalberg, E. (1978). *J. Neurochem.* **31**, 5–11.

Helenius, A. and Simons, K. (1977) *Proc Natl. Acad. Sci.* **74**, 529–532.

Helle, K. B., Fillenz, M., Stanford, C., Pihl, K. E. and Srebro, B. (1979). *J. Neurochem.* **32**, 1351–1355.

Hino, Y., Asano, A. and Sato, R. (1978). *J. Biochem.* **83**, 925–934.

Hizi, A. and Yagil, G. (1974). *Eur. J. Biochem.* **45**, 211–221.

Hoeldtke, R. and Kaufman, S. (1977). *J. Biol. Chem.* **252**, 3160–3169.

Hökfelt, T., Fuxe, K. and Goldstein, M. (1973). *Brain Res.* **62**, 461–469.

Hökfelt, T., Fuxe, K., Goldstein, M. and Johansson, O. (1974). *Brain Res.* **66**, 235–251.

Hökfelt, T., Elde, R., Johansson, O., Luft, R. and Arimura, A. (1975). *Neurosci. L.* **1**, 231–235.

Holland, P. C. and MacLennan, D. H. (1976). *J. Biol. Chem.* **251**, 2030–2036.

Hopff, W. H., Riggio, G. and Waser, P. G. (1975) *In* "Cholinergic Mechanisms" (P. G. Waser, ed.). Raven Press, New York.

Hopgood, M. F., Ballard, F. J., Reshef, L. and Hanson, R. W. (1973). *Biochem. J.* **134**, 445–453.

Hörtnagl, H., Winkler, H. and Lochs, H. (1973). *J. Neurochem.* **20**, 977–985.

Houdebine, L.-M. (1976). *Eur. J. Biochem.* **68**, 219–225.

Houdebine, L.-M. and Gaye, P. (1976). *Eur. J. Biochem.* **63**, 9–14.

Houslay, M. D. and Tipton, K. F. (1973). *Biochem. J.* **135**, 173–186.

Hudson, L and Hay, F. C. (1976). "Practical Immunology". Blackwood, Oxford, England.

Hunter, W. M. (1967). *In* "Handbook of Experimental Immunology", (D. M. Weir, Ed.), pp. 608–654. Blackwell, Oxford.

Hyden, H. (1973). *In* "Macromolecules and Behaviour" (G. B. Ansell and P. D. Bradley, Eds), pp. 3–26. Macmillans, London.

Ikehara, Y., Takahashi, K., Mansho, K., Eto, S. and Kato, K. (1977). *Biochim. Biophys. Acta* **470**, 202–211.

Jean, D. H. and Albers, R. W. (1976). *Biochim. Biophys. Acta* **452**, 219–226.

Jensen, K. (1959). Thesis, Munksgaard, Copenhagen.

Johnston, J. P. (1968). *Biochem. Pharmacol.* **17**, 1285–1297.

Jonsson, S. and Kronvall, G. (1974). *Eur. J. Immunol.* **4**, 29–33.

Jørgensen, O. S. (1976). *J. Neurochem.* **27**, 1223–1227.

Jørgensen, O. S. (1977). *FEBS Letts,* **79,** 42–44.

Jørgensen, A. O., Subrahmanyan, L., Turnbull, C. and Kalnins, V. I. (1976). *Proc. Natl. Acad. Sci.* **73,** 3129–3196.

Kabat, E. A. (1967). *In* "Methods in Immunology and Immunochemistry" Vol. 1, (C. A. Williams and M. W. Chase, Eds) pp. 335–339. Academic Press, New York and London.

Kabat, E. A. (1971). "Kabat and Mayers Experimental Immunochemistry", 3rd Ed., pp. 89–90. Charles C. Thomas, Springfield, Ill.

Kan, K. S. K., Chao, L. P. and Eng, L. F. (1978). *Brain Res.* **146,** 221–229.

Kao, I. and Drachman, D. B. (1977). *Science* **196,** 527–529.

Kaplan, G., Unkeless, J.C. and Cotin, Z. A. (1979). *Proc. Natl. Acad. Sci.* **76,** 3824–3828.

Karlin, A., Holtzman, E., Valderrama, R., Damle, V., Hsu, K. and Reyes, F. (1978). *J. Cell Biology* **76,** 577–592.

Karlsson, E., Heilbronn, E. and Widlund, L. (1972). *FEBS Lett* **28,** 107–111.

Katan, M. B., Van Harten-Loosebroek, N. and Groot, G. S. P. (1976). *Eur. J. Biochem.* **70,** 409–417.

Kessler, S. W. (1975). *J. Immunol.* **115,** 1617–1624.

Kessler, S. W. (1976). *J. Immunol.* **117,** 1482–1490.

Koch, C. and Nielsen, H. E. (1975). *Scand. J. Immunol.* **4,** Suppl. 2, 121–124.

Köhler, G. and Milstein, C. (1975). *Nature* **256,** 495–497.

Köhler, G. and Milstein, C. (1976). *Eur. J. Immunol.* **6,** 511–519.

Kostner, G. and Holasek, A. (1972). *Anal. Biochem.* **46,** 680–683.

Kraehenbuhl, J. P., de Grandi, P. B. and Campiche, M. A. (1971). *J. Cell. Biol.* **50,** 432–445.

Kristiansen, T. (1976). *In* "Immunoadsorbents in Protein Purification", E. Ruoslahti, Ed.), pp. 19–27. Universitetsforlaget, Oslo.

Krohn, K. A., Knight, L. C., Harwig, J. F. and Welch, M. J. (1977). *Biochim. Biophys. Acta* **490,** 497–505.

Krøll, J. (1973a). *In* "A Manual of Quantitative Immunoelectrophoresis", (N. H. Axelsen, J. Krøll and B. Weeke, Eds), pp. 57–59. Universitetsforlaget, Oslo.

Krøll, J. (1973b). *In* "A Manual of Quantitative Immunoelectrophoresis, (N. H. Axelsen, J. Krøll and B. Weeke, Eds), pp. 79–81. Universitetsforlaget, Oslo.

Kronvall, G. and Frommel, D. (1970). *Immunochem.* **7,** 124–127.

Kronvall, G., Seal, U. S., Finstad, J. and Williams, R. C. Jr. (1970). *J. Immunol.* **104,** 140–147.

Kuma, F., Prough, R. A. and Masters, B. S. S. (1976). *Arch. Biochem. Biophys.* **172,** 600–607.

Kwapinski, J. B. G. (1972). "Methodology of Immunochemical and Immunological Research", pp. 286–306. Wiley-Interscience, New York.

Kyte, J. (1976). *J. Cell Biol.* **68,** 287–303.

Lagercrantz, H. (1976). *Neuroscience* **1,** 81–92.

Landon, J., Livanon, J. and Greenwood, F. C. (1967). *Biochem. J.* **105,** 1075–1083.

Lanzerotti, R. H. and Gullino, P. M. (1972). *Anal. Biochem.* **50,** 344–353.

Larsson, L. I., Fahrenkrug, J. and Schaffalitzky de Muckadell, O. B. (1977). *Science* **197,** 1374–1375.

Laurell, C.-B. (1966). *Anal. Biochem.* **15,** 45–52.

Lazarides, E. (1976). *J. Cell Biol.* **68,** 202–219.

Lee, L. D., Baden, H. P. and Cheng, C. K. (1978). *J. Immunol. Meths.* **24**, 155–162.

Lee, T.-C., Baker, R. C., Stephens, N. and Snyder, F. (1977). *Biochim. Biophys. Acta* **489**, 25–31.

Leek, A. E. and Chard, T. (1974). *In:* "L'Alpha Foetoproteine", (R. Masseyeff, Ed.). INSERM, Paris.

Levin, W., Lu, A. Y. H., Thomas, P. E., Ryan, D., Kizer, D. E. and Griffin, M. J. (1978). *Proc. Natl. Acad. Sci.* **75**, 3240–3243.

Levine, L. (1967). Imunochemical appproaches to the study of the nervous system. *In* "The Neurosciences" (G. C. Quarton, T. Melneckuk and F. O. Schmitt, Eds). Rockerfeller Universal Res., New York.

Lin, L.-F. Y., Clejan, L. and Beattie, D. S. (1978). *Eur. J. Biochem.* **87**, 171–179.

Lind, I. and Mansa, B. (1968). *Acta. Pathol. Microbiol. Scand.* (B) **73**, 637–645.

Lind, I., Live, I. and Mansa, B. (1970). *Acta. Pathol. Microbiol. Scand.* (B) **78**, 673–682.

Ling, C. M. and Overby, L. R. (1972). *J. Immunol.* **109**, 834–841.

Littlefield, J. W. (1964). *Science* **145**, 709–710.

Loft, H. (1975). *Scand. J. Immunol.* **4**, Suppl. 2, 115–119.

Loh, Y. P. (1979). *Proc. Natl. Acad. Sci.* **76**, 796–800.

Louvard, D., Semeriva, M. and Maroux, S. (1976a). *J. Mol. Biol.* **106**, 1023–1035.

Louvard, D., Vannier, Ch., Maroux, S., Pages, J.-M. and Ladunski, C. (1976b). *Anal. Biochem.* **76**, 83–94.

Lowe, C. R. and Dean, P. D. G. (1974). "Affinity Chromatography" Wiley, London.

Lundahl, P. and Liljas, L. (1975). *Anal. Biochem.* **65**, 50–59.

Luzio, J. P., Newby, A. C. and Hales, C. N. (1976). *Biochem. J.* **154**, 11–21.

Malthe-Sørenssen, D., Eskeland, T. and Fonnum, F. (1973). *Brain Res.* **62**, 517–522.

Malthe-Sørenssen, D., Lea, T., Fonnum, F. and Eskeland, T. (1978). *J. Neurochem.* **30**, 35–46.

Mancini, G., Carbonara, A. O. and Hereman, S. J. F. (1965). *Immunochemistry* **2**, 235–254.

Manning, R., Dils, R. and Mayer, R. J. (1976). *Biochem. J.* **153**, 463–468.

Marchesi, V. T. and Furthmayr, H. (1976). *Ann. Rev. Biochem.* **45**, 667–698.

Marengo, T. S., Harrison, R., Lunt, G. G. and Behan, P. O. (1979). *Lancet* **1**, 442.

Mason, T. L., Poyton, R. O., Wharton, D. C. and Schatz, G. (1973). *J. Biol. Chem.* **248**, 1346–1354.

Matsura, S., Fujii-Kuriyama, Y. and Toshiro, Y. (1978). *J. Cell. Biol.* **78**, 503–519.

Maurer, P. M. (1971). *In* "Methods in Immunology and Immunochemistry", Vol. III, (C. A. Williams and M. W. Chase, Eds), pp. 1–58. Academic Press, New York and London.

McCans, J. L., Lane, L. K., Lindenmayer, G. E., Butler, V. P. Jr. and Schwartz, A. (1974). *Proc. Natl. Acad. Sci.* **71**, 2249–2452.

McCans, J. L., Lindenmayer, G. E., Pitts, B. J. R., Ray, M. W., Rayner, B. D., Butler, V. P. Jr. and Schwartz, A. (1975). *J. Biol. Chem.* **250**, 7257–7265.

McCauley, R. and Racker, E. (1973). Separation of two monoamine oxidase S from Bovine brain. *Mol. Cell. Biochem.* **1**, 73–81.

McLaughlin, B. J., Wood, J. G., Saito, K., Roberts, E. and Wu, J. (1975). *Brain Res.* **85**, 355–371.

McNeil, T. H. and Sladek, J. R. (1978). *Science,* **200**, 72–74.

Miles, L. E. M. and Hales, C. N. (1968a). *Nature* **219**, 186–189.

Miles, L. E. M. and Hales, C. N. (1968b). *Biochem. J.* **108,** 611–618.
Minamuira, N. and Yasunobu, K. T. (1978). *Arch. Biochem. Biophys.* **189,** 481–489.
Mitchison, N. A. (1968). *Immunology* **15,** 509–530.
Moody, G. J. (1976). *Lab. Pract.* **25,** 575–581.
Moorman, A. F. M., Grivell, L. A., Lamie, F. and Smits, H. L. (1978). *Biochim. Biophys. Acta* **518,** 351–365.
Morgan, J. L., Rodkey, L. S. and Spooner, B. S. (1977). *Science* **197,** 578–580.
Morimoto, T., Matsura, S., Sasaki, S., Tashiro, Y. and Omura, T. (1976). *J. Cell. Biol.* **68,** 189–201.
Murphy, M. J. (1976). *Biochem. J.* **159,** 287–292.
Nagatsu, I. and Kando, Y. (1975). *Act. Hist. Cyt.* **8,** 279–287.
Nicklin, M. G. and Stephen, J. (1974). *Immunochem.* **11,** 35–40.
Niemi, W. D., Nastuk, W. L., Chang, H. W., Penn, A. S. and Rosenberg, T. L. (1979). *Exp. Neurol.* **63,** 1–27.
Nilsson, G., Said, S. and Goldstein, M. (1978). *Brain Res.* **155,** 239–248.
Nisonoff, A. and Palmer, J. L. (1964). *Science* **143,** 376.
Norrild, B., Bjerrum, O. J. and Vestergaard, B. F. (1977). *Anal. Biochem.* **81,** 432–441.
Noshiro, M. and Omura, T. (1978). *J. Biochem.* **83,** 61–77.
Oesch, F. and Bentley, P. (1976). *Nature* **259,** 53–55.
O'Farrell, P. H. (1975). *J. Biol. Chem.* **250,** 4007–4021.
Okayasu, T., Onon, T. and Shinojima, K. (1977). *Lipids* **12,** 267–271.
Olden, K. and Yamada, K. M. (1977). *Anal. Biochem.* **78,** 483–490.
Olsen, R. W., Meunier, J.-C. and Changeux, J.-P. (1972). *FEBS Letts* **28,** 96–100.
Orlov, G. E. and Gurvich, A. E. (1971) in *Kongr. Mikrobiol. Mater. Kongr. Mikrobiol. Bulg. 2nd 1969* (I. Pashev, Ed.) Vol. 1, 225–229.
Ouchterlony, O. (1968). *In* "Handbook of Immunodiffusion and Immunoelectric-phoresis", Ann-Arbor Science Publ., Ann Arbor.
Owen, P. and Smyth, C. J. (1977). *In* "Immunochemistry of Enzymes and their antibodies" (M. R. J. Salton, Ed.). Wiley, London.
Pages, J.-M., Varenne, S. and Lazdunski, C. (1976). *Eur. J. Biochem.* **67,** 145–153.
Palacios, R., Palmiter, R. D. and Schimke, R. T. (1972). *J. Biol. Chem.* **247,** 2316–2321.
Papermaster, B. W., Sordahl, L. A. and Stene, H. L. (1976). *In* "Non Isotopic Immunoassays". Conference Handbook. Robert S. First, Inc.
Paskin, N. and Mayer, R. J. (1976). *Biochem. J.* **159,** 181–184.
Patrick, J. and Lindstrom, J. (1973). Science **180,** 871–872.
Peavy, D. E. and Hansen, R. J. (1975). *Biochem. Biophys. Res. Commun.* **66,** 1106–1111.
Philippidis, H., Hansen, R. W., Reshef, L., Hopgood, M. F. and Ballard, F. J. (1972). *Biochem. J.* **126,** 1127–1134.
Piazzi, S. E. (1969). *Anal. Biochem.* **27,** 281–284.
Pickel, V. M., Tong, H. J. and Reis, D. J. (1975). *Proc. Nat. Acad. Sci.* **72,** 659–663.
Poole, A. R. (1974). "Immunological methods for the study of the cellular localization of proteins in Biochemistry", Vol. 4. Subcellular Studies, Longman, London.
Porath, J. and Sundberg, L. (1970). *Protides Biol. Fluids* **18,** 401–407.
Porath, J., Aspberg, K., Drevin, H. and Axen, R. (1973). *J. Chromatog.* **86,** 53–56.

Poyton, R. O. and Schatz, G. (1975). *J. Biol. Chem.* **250**, 762–766.
Price, M. R. and Baldwin, R. W. (1977). "Cell Surface Reviews," Vol. 1. (G. Post and G. Nicholson, Eds) Elsevier, Amsterdam.
Prough, R. A. and Ziegler, D. M. (1977). *Arch. Biochem. Biophys.* **180**, 363–373.
Raftell, M., Berzins, K. and Blomberg, F. (1977). *Arch. Biochim. Biophys.* **181**, 534–541.
Readhead, C., Addison, G. M., Hales, C. W. and Letimann, H. (1973). *J. Endocr.* **59**, 313–323.
Reed, K., Vandlen, R. L., Bode, J., Duguid, J. K. and Raftery, M. A. (1975). *Arch. Biochem. Biophys.* **167**, 138–144.
Reis, D. J., Pickel, V. M., Shikimi, T. and Joh, T. H. (1975). *Trans. Amer. Soc. Neurochem.* **6**, 155.
Remacle, J., Fowler, S., Beaufay, H., Amarcostesec, A. and Berthet, J. (1976). *J. Cell. Biol.* **71**, 551–564.
Remacle, J., Fowler, S., Beaufay, H. and Berthet, J. (1974). *J. Cell. Biol.* 237–240.
Remy, M. H. and Poznasky, M. J. (1978). *Lancet* July 8th, 68–70.
Rhoads, R. E., McKnight, G. S. and Schmike, R. T. (1973). *J. Biol. Chem.* **248**, 2031–2039.
Rice, R. H. and Means, G. E. (1971). *J. Biol. Chem.* **246**, 831–832.
Rieger, F., Bon, S., Massoulie, J., Cartaud, J., Picard, B. and Benda, P. (1976). *Eur. J. Biochem.* **68**, 513–521.
Roberts, R. and Painter, A. (1977). *Biochim. Biophys. Acta* **480**, 521–526.
Roisen, F., Inczedy-Marcsek, M., Hsu, L. and Yorke, W. (1978). *Science* **199**, 1445–1448.
Rosen, J. M., Woo, S. L. C. and Comstock, J. P. (1975). *Biochemistry* **14**, 2895–2903.
Rosenberry, T. L. and Richardson, J. M. (1977). *Biochemistry* **16**, 3550–3558.
Ross, E. and Schatz, G. (1976). J. Biol. Chem. **251**, 1997–2004.
Ross, R. A., Joh, T. H. and Reis, D. J. (1978). *J. Neurochem.* **31**, 1491–1500.
Rossier, J. (1975). *Brain Res.* **98**, 619–622.
Rossier, J. (1976a). *J. Neurochem.* **26**, 543–548.
Rossier, J. (1976b). *J. Neurochem.* **26**, 549–553.
Rossier, J., Bauman, A., Rieger, F. and Benda, P. (1975) *In* "Cholinergic Mechanisms" (P. G. Waser, Ed.) pp. 283–292. Raven Press, New York.
Rothman, J. E. and Lenard, J. (1977). *Science* **195**, 743–753.
Ruoslahti, E. (1976). *In* "Immunoadsorbents in Protein Purification, (E. Ruoslahti, Ed.), pp. 3–7, Universitetsforlaget, Oslo.
Rush, R. A., Costa, M., Furness, J. B. and Geffen, L. B. (1976). *Neurosci. Lett* **3**, 209–213.
Russell, S., Davey, J. and Mayer, R. J., (1978a). *Proc. Europ. Soc. Neurochem.* **1**, 544.
Russell, S., Davey, J. and Mayer, R. J. (1978b). *Proc. Europ. Soc. Neurochem.* **1**, 545.
Ryan, D. E., Thomas, P. E. and Levin, W. (1977). *Mol. Pharmacol.* **13**, 521–532.
Saito, K. (1978). *Fol. Pharm. J.* **74**, 427–440.
Salvaterra, P. M. and Mahler, H. R. (1976). *J. Biol. Chem.* **251**, 6327–6334.
Sandler, M. and Youdim, M. B. H. (1972). *Pharmacol. Rev.* **24**, 331–348.
Schimke, R. T., Sweeney, E. W. and Berlin, C. M. (1965). *J. Biol. Chem.* **240**, 322–331.
Schlaepfer, W. W. (1977). J. Cell. Biol. **74**, 226–240.

Schmidt. J. and Raftery, M. A. (1973). Biochemistry **12**, 852–856.
Schmitt, M., Rittinghaus, K., Scheurich, P., Schwulera, U. and Dose, K. (1978). *Biochim. Biophys. Acta* **509**, 410–418.
Schultzberg, M., Dreyfus, C. F., Gershon, M. D., Hökfelt, T., Elde, R. P. Nilsson, G., Said, S., and Goldstein, M. (1978). *Brain Res.* **155** 239–248.
Schutlzberg, M., Hökfelt, T., Terenius, L., Brandt, J., Elde, R. P. and Goldstein, M. (1979). *Neuroscience* **4**, 249–270.
Sewell, M. M. H. (1967). *Science Tools* **14**, 11–12.
Sherline, P. and Schiarone, K. (1977). *Science* **198**, 1038–1040.
Shuster, L. and O'Toole, C. (1974). *Life Sci.* **15**, 645–656.
Singer, S. J., Ash, J. F., Bourguignon, L. Y. W., Heggeness, M. H. and Louvard, D. (1978). *J. Supram. Struct.* **9**, 373–389.
Singh, V. K. and McGreer, P. L. (1974). *Life Sci.* **15**, 901–913.
Smith, J. A., Hurrell, J. G. R. and Leach, S. J. (1978). *Anal. Biochem.* **87**, 299–305.
Sobel, A., Weber, M. and Changeux, J.-P. (1977). *Eur. J. Biochem.* **80**, 215–224.
Söderholm, C. J., Smyth, C. J. and Wadström, T. (1975). *Scand. J. Immunol.* **4**, Suppl. 2, 107–113.
Speake, B. K., Dils, R. and Mayer, R. J. (1975). *Biochem. J.* **148**, 309–320.
Speake, B. K., Dils, R. and Mayer, R. J. (1976). *Biochem. J.* **154**, 359–370.
Spector, S., Felix, A., Semenuk, G. and Finberg, J. P. M. (1978). *J. Neurochem.* **30**, 685–689.
Stadler, H. and Tashiro, T. (1978). *Proc. Eur. Soc. Neurochem.* **1**, 580.
Stanley, E. F. and Drachman, D. B. (1978). *Science* **200**, 1285–1287.
Stansbie, D., Denton, R. M., Bridges, B. J., Pask, H. T. and Randle, P. J. (1976). *Biochem. J.* 225–236.
Steiner, A. L. (1974). *Meths. in Enzymol.* **38**, 96–105.
Stephen, R. E. (1975). *Anal. Biochem.* **69**, 369–379.
Stephenson, G. T. (1974). *Nature* **247**, 477–478.
Sternberger, L. A. (1974). "Immunocytochemistry. Prentice Hall, New Jersey.
Sternberger, L. A., Hardy, P. H., Cuculis, J. J. and Meyer, H. G. (1970). *J. Histochem. Cytochem.* **18**, 315–333.
Strange, P. G. (1978). *Biochem. J.* **176**, 583–590.
Strauss, A. W., Alberts, A. W., Hennessy, S. and Vagelos, P. R. (1975). *Proc. Natl. Acad. Sci. USA* **72**, 4366–4370.
Sugiyama, H., Benda, P., Meunier, J.-C. and Changeux, J.-P. (1973). *FEBS Lett.* **35**, 124–128.
Suttie, J. W., Carlisle, T. L. and Cranfield, L. (1977) *In* "Calcium-Binding Proteins and Calcium Function" (R. H. Kretsinger, D. H. MacLennan and F. L. Siegel Eds). N. Holland Publ. Co., New York.
Svendsen, P. J. (1973). *Scand. J. Immunol.* **4**, Suppl. 1, 69–70.
Swaab, D. F. and Fisser, B. (1977). *Neuroscience Lett.* **7**, 313–317.
Takesue, Y. and Nishi, Y. (1976). *J. Biochem.* **79**, 479–488.
Takesue, Y. and Nishi, Y. (1978). *J. Membrane Biol.* **39**, 285–296.
Takesue, S. and Omura, T. (1970). *Biochem. Biophys. Res. Comm.* **40**, 369–377.
Tashiro, T. and Stadler, H. (1978). *Eur. J. Biochem.* **90**, 479–487.
Teichberg, V. I., Sobel, A. and Changeux, J.-P. (1977). *Nature* **267**, 540–542.
Ternynck, T. and Avrameas, S. (1976). *In* "Immunoadsorbents in Protein Purification", (E. Ruoslahti, Ed.), pp. 29–35. Universitetsforlaget, Oslo.
The, T. H. and Feltkamp, T. E. W. (1970). *Immunology,* **18**, 875–881.
Thomas, P. E., Lu, A. Y. H., Ryan, D., West, S. B., Kawalek, J. and Levin, W.

(1976). *Mol. Pharmacol.* **12**, 746–758.

Thomas, P. E., Lu, A. Y. H., West, S. B., Ryan, D., Miwa, G. T. and Levin, W. (1977). *Mol. Pharmacol.* **13**, 819–831.

Tipton, K. F., Houslay, M. D. and Mantle, T. J. (1976). *In* "Monoamine Oxidase and its Inhibition", Ciba Found. Sym. **39**, (New Series) pp. 5–33. Elsevier, North Holland, Amsterdam.

Tripathi, R. K. and O'Brien, R. D. (1977). *Biochim. Biophys. Acta* **480**, 382–389.

Tsuji, S., Rieger, F., Peltre, G., Massoulie, J. and Benda, P. (1972). *J. Neurochem.* **19**, 989–997.

Uhl, G. R., Goodman, R. R., Kuhar, M. J., Childers, S. R. and Snyder, S. H. (1979). *Brain Res.* **166**, 75–94.

Unsicker, K., Drenckhahn, D. Gröschel-Stewart, U., Schumacher, U. and (1978). Cell Tissue Res. **188**, 341–344.

Uriel, J. (1964). *In* "Immunoelectrophoretic Analysis". (P. Grabar and Burtin Eds), Elsevier, Holland.

Valderrama, R., Weill, C. L., McNamee, M. and Karlin, A. (1976). *Ann. N.Y. Acad. Sci. USA,* **274**, 108–115.

Vannier, Ch., Louvard, D., Maroux, S. and Desnuelle, P. (1976). *Biochim. Biophys. Acta* **455**, 185–199.

Walker, J. H. and Mayer, R. J. (1976). *Biochem. Soc. Trans.* **4**, 342–344.

Walker, J. H. and Mayer, R. J. (1977). *Biochem. Soc. Trans.* **5**, 1101–1103.

Walker, J. H., Betts, S. A., Manning, R. and Mayer, R. J. (1976). *Biochem. J.* **159**, 355–362.

Watson, S. J., Richard, C. W. and Barchas, J. D. (1978). *Science* **200**, 1180–1182.

Webb, K. S., Mickey, D. D., Stove, K. R. and Paulson, D. F. (1977). *J. Immun. Methods.* **14**, 343–353.

Weeke, B. (1973a). *In* "A Manual of Quantitative Immunoelectrophoresis", pp. 37–46. Universitetsforlaget, Oslo.

Weeke, B. (1973b). *In* "A Manual of Quantitative Immunoelectrophoresis, (N. H. Axelsen, J. Krøll and B. Weeke, Eds), pp. 47–56. Universitetsforlaget, Oslo.

Werner, S. (1974). *Eur. J. Biochem.* **43**, 39–48.

Werner, S. and Machleidt, W. (1978). *Eur. J. Biochem.* **90**, 99–105.

Whittaker, V. P. (1977). *Naturwissenschaften* **64**, 606–611.

Williams, C. A. and Chase, M. W. (1967). *In* "Methods in Immunology and Immunochemistry", Vol. 1, pp. 307–335. Academic Press, New York and London.

Williams, C. A. and Schupf, N. (1977). *Science* **196**, 328–330.

Winkler, H. (1976). *Neuroscience* **1**, 65–80.

Winkler, H. (1977). *Neuroscience* **2**, 657–683.

Winkler, H., Schneider, F. H., Rufener, C., Nakane, P. K. and Hortnagl, H. (1974). *In* "Advances in Cytopharmacol Vol. 2, (B. Ceccarelli, F. Clements and J. Meldolesi, Eds), pp. 127–139. Raven Press, New York.

Witzemann, V. and Raftery, M. A. (1978). *Biochem. Biophys. Res. Comm.* **85**, 623–631.

Woodhead, J. S., Addison, G. M. and Hales, C. N. (1974). *Br. Med. Bull.* **30**, 44–49.

Wooten, G. F., Park, D. H., Joh, T. H. and Reis, D. J. (1978). *Nature* **275**, 324–325.

Yalow, R. S. (1978). *Science* **200**, 1236–1245.

Zomzely-Neurath, C. and Keller, A. (1977). *Neurochem. Res.* **2**, 353–377.

Subject Index

Figure numbers in **bold** refer to sections discussing the indexed term